LB
1588
U6
H86
1993

Humphrey, James
Harry, 1911-
Elementary school
child health

DATE DUE

ELEMEN   **LTH**

AUDREY COHEN COLLEGE LIBRARY
75 Varick St. 12th Floor
New York, NY 10013

ABOUT THE AUTHOR

James H. Humphrey, Professor Emeritus at the University of Maryland, has published over 60 books and 200 articles and research reports. One of America's leading health educators over the last half century, he has been a consultant to numerous school systems throughout the country in the development of school health programs. In addition to being a former Research Editor for the *Journal of School Health,* Dr. Humphrey was a charter member and first chairman elect of the Research Council of the American School Health Association.

ELEMENTARY SCHOOL CHILD HEALTH

For Parents and Teachers

By

JAMES H. HUMPHREY, ED.D.
Professor Emeritus
University of Maryland

With a Foreword by
Michael J. Schaffer

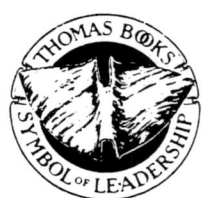

CHARLES C THOMAS • PUBLISHER
Springfield • Illinois • U.S.A.

Published and Distributed Throughout the World by
CHARLES C THOMAS • PUBLISHER
2600 South First Street
Springfield, Illinois 62794-9265

This book is protected by copyright. No part of
it may be reproduced in any manner without
written permission from the publisher.

© *1993 by* CHARLES C THOMAS • PUBLISHER
ISBN 0-398-05868-7
Library of Congress Catalog Card Number: 93-3627

With THOMAS BOOKS *careful attention is given to all details of manufacturing and design. It is the Publisher's desire to present books that are satisfactory as to their physical qualities and artistic possibilities and appropriate for their particular use.* THOMAS BOOKS *will be true to those laws of quality that assure a good name and good will.*

Printed in the United States of America
SC-R-3

Library of Congress Cataloging-in-Publication Data

Humphrey, James Harry, 1911–
    Elementary school child health : for parents and teachers / by James H. Humphrey ; with a foreword by Michael J. Schaffer.
      p.   cm.
    Includes bibliographical references and index.
    ISBN 0-398-05868-7
    1. Health education (Elementary) – United States. 2. Children – Health and hygiene – Study and teaching (Elementary) – United States.
3. Education, Elementary – United States – Activity programs.
I. Title.
LB1588.U6H86   1993
372.3'7'0973 – dc20   93-3627
                                                                                                     CIP

FOREWORD

Ever since the one-room school opened for business, and the first teacher admonished her students to wash their hands before eating lunch, health education has been a part of the school curriculum.

Over the years, America has been fortunate to lead the world in the quality of its health education. Hardly a year has passed without the discovery of a long-sought-after cure or treatment for a disease or major information about how to maintain one's health. A very broad discipline, health includes physical, social, and emotional elements as well as nutrition, fitness, growth and development, disease prevention, mental and personal health. We must all address these areas of concern. This is not such an easy task, however. A mountain of information exists today that should be incorporated into our daily lives.

The primary health educators of all children are their parents. Sadly, very few parents ever receive any formal training in health education. Parents are expected to "just know everything there is to know about health and how to teach it to their kids." After parents, the secondary health educators of all children are their teachers. They too are expected to be omnicient when it comes to health. Unfortunately, they, too, seldom receive any more formal training than the typical parent.

Learning about health can be a difficult and time-consuming task. Although much information is available through various forms of media—newspapers, radio, television, magazines, journals, and electronic data bases—it is often fragmentary and scattered and sometimes can be misleading or unsubstantiated. Parents and teachers may become frustrated in their search for accurate health information or lack the time necessary to research properly.

Fortunately, Professor Humphrey's book provides an excellent resource for those of us interested in child and school health. This one volume pulls together an extraordinary amount of useful information. It contains everything that a parent or teacher needs to know about health of children between the ages of five and twelve. Professor Humphrey's work is based on a lifetime of experience as a professional health educator. His comprehensive approach is accurate, up-to-date, and on the forefront of health education. He provides expert advice and imparts his wisdom in a clear and concise manner.

Michael J. Schaffer
Supervisor of Health Education, K–12
Prince George's County Public Schools
Upper Marlboro, Maryland

PREFACE

Herbert Hoover, the thirty-first president of the United States, is credited with the oft-quoted statement: "Children are our most valuable natural resource." Of course, this is undeniably so. Therefore, there should be no doubt about the importance of child health.

This book has been prepared for parents and teachers who have the wherewithal to provide the guidance necessary to promote the health of children of elementary school age.

The introductory chapter describes such terms as health, health knowledge, attitudes, and practices, health education, and fitness.

Chapters 2, 3, and 4 are concerned with the physical, social, and emotional health of children. Taken into account are such factors as needs of children, teacher observation of health of children, and how children can develop physical, social, and emotional health concepts.

Nutrition is the subject of Chapter 5 and considers eating habits of children and childhood obesity. In chapter 6 emphasis is placed on body restoration in the form of rest, sleep, and relaxation.

In Chapter 7 the area of stress is discussed as an impact on child health with emphasis on home and family stress and stress in the school environment.

The final chapter is concerned with the elementary school health program and takes into account such areas as school health service, healthful school living and school health education.

CONTENTS

	Page
Foreword	v
Preface	vii

Chapter

1. THE MEANING OF HEALTH AND RELATED TERMS 3

    The Meaning of Health . . . Health Knowledge, Attitudes, and Practice . . . The Meaning of Health Education . . . The Meaning of Fitness

2. PHYSICAL HEALTH OF CHILDREN 14

    Child Health in Relation to Physical Growth and Development . . . Teacher Observation of the Physical Health of Children . . . Helping Children Learn About the Human Organism . . . Physical Activity and Exercise for Children . . . Types of Physical Activities and Exercises for Children . . . School Physical Activity Programs . . . Out-of-School Physical Activity Programs . . . Current Status of Physical Fitness of Children . . . Helping Children Learn About Physical Activity and Exercise

3. EMOTIONAL HEALTH OF CHILDREN 44

    Factors Concerning Emotional Health . . . Emotional Needs of Children . . . Some Guidelines for the Emotional Health of Children . . . Opportunities for Improving Emotional Health in the School Environment . . . Teacher Observation of the Emotional Health of Children . . . Helping Children Learn About Emotional Health

4. SOCIAL HEALTH OF CHILDREN 63

    Social Needs of Children . . . Guidelines for Social Health . . . Implications of Research in Social Behavior of Children . . . Evaluating Contributions of School Experiences to Social Health . . . Helping Children Learn About Social Health

5. NUTRITION AND CHILD HEALTH 76

    Nutrition . . . Diet . . . Children's Eating Habits . . . Childhood Obesity . . . Helping Children Learn About Foods and Nutrition

6. BODY RESTORATION AND CHILD HEALTH 98
   Fatigue . . . Rest . . . Sleep . . . Children's Sleep Habits . . . Relaxation . . . The Meaning of Relaxation and Related Terms . . . Learning how to Relax . . . Progressive Relaxation . . . Using Relaxation with Children . . . Mental Practice and Imagery in Relaxation . . . Helping Children Learn About Rest, Sleep, and Relaxation
7. STRESS AND CHILD HEALTH 118
   The Meaning of Stress . . . The Concept of Stress . . . Home and Family Stress . . . School Stress
8. THE ELEMENTARY SCHOOL HEALTH PROGRAM 137

Afterword 143
Bibliography 145
Index 147

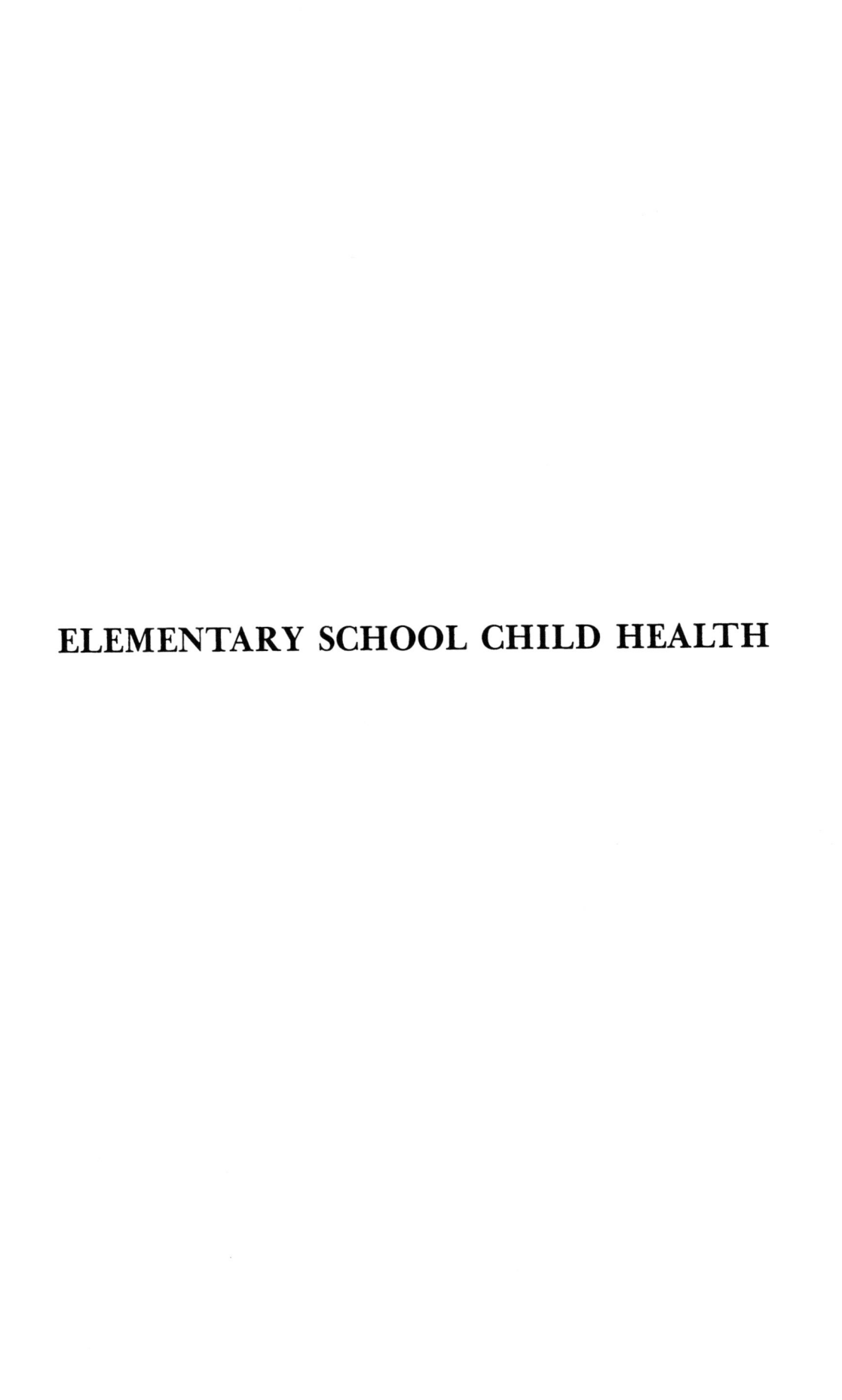

ELEMENTARY SCHOOL CHILD HEALTH

Chapter 1

THE MEANING OF HEALTH AND RELATED TERMS

An intelligent discussion and the sound treatment of any subject should perhaps begin with some sort of understanding of the terminology connected with that particular subject. This implies a consistent use of carefully defined terms as well as an insight into the relationship between certain terms. The many attempts to develop new definitions of old terms and the introduction of new terms in certain fields have resulted, in some instances, in widespread confusion in the meaning and relationship of various commonly-used terms in these various fields. This widespread confusion in terminology exists in the area of *health.* I say this because I have had many inquiries over the years from parents and teachers with reference to the meaning of health and related terms. Such questions as "What is really meant by good health?" and "Just what does it mean to be fit?" seem to make it appropriate to devote a somewhat detailed discussion to this subject. To this end, the following terms will be described in the ensuing discussions: *health, health knowledge, health attitudes, health practice, health education,* and *fitness* (physical, social, emotional, and intellectual).

THE MEANING OF HEALTH

Throughout the ages various scholars and philosophers have made pronouncements depicting the importance and meaning of health. Two examples of such citations are presented here: In 300 BC the the Greek anatomist Herophilus, personal physician to Alexander the Great, postulated that when *health is absent, wisdom cannot reveal itself, art cannot become manifest, strength cannot fight, wealth becomes useless, and intelligence cannot be applied.* Centuries later, Arthur Schopenhauer (1788–1860), a German philosopher, proclaimed, *If you must waste money, time and health, do so in that order.*

In modern times, the precise meaning that one associates with the term *health* depends in a large measure on the particular frame of reference in which it is used. In recent years it was a relatively common practice to think of health in terms of the condition of the living organism that functioned normally. This idea about health is one that is still accepted by many people. In subscribing to this particular concept, these individuals tend to think of health predominantly as a state in which there is absence of pain or symptoms related to a poorly functioning organism. When thought of only in this manner, health is considered primarily in terms of a state in which there is absence of disease.

A modern concept considers health more and more in terms of *well-being*, which is perhaps the most important human value. In considering health from a point of view of well-being, the ideal state of health would be one in which all of the various parts of the human organism function at an optimum level at all times. This perhaps is what the notable American author and editor H. L. Mencken meant many years ago when he characterized the healthy man as one perfectly adjusted to his environment. Although it is very unlikely that the human organism will ever achieve the ideal state suggested here, such a level is ordinarily used as a standard for diagnosing or appraising the human health status.

The old meaning of health that considered it primarily only in terms of absence of disease tended to place it in a negative sense. The more modern concept places more positive emphasis on the term. This is to say that the meaning of health is interpreted as a level of well-being as well. It seems logical to assume that modern society's goal should be in the direction of achieving the highest level of well-being for all of its citizens, children as well as adults.

HEALTH KNOWLEDGE, ATTITUDES, AND PRACTICE

Any discussion of health should consider the three important aspects of health knowledge, health attitudes, and health practice. Each of these dimensions will be dealt with separately, but it appears important at the outset to consider them together for the purpose of a better understanding of how they are related.

In order to benefit most from health learning experiences, it is most important that these experiences develop into desirable health practices. Thus, the ultimate goal should be in the direction of a kind of behavior that will be likely to insure optimum present and future health for the individual. However, before the most desirable and worthwhile health practices can be achieved, there is a need for a certain amount of desirable health knowledge, along with a proper attitude, in making appropriate application of the knowledge to health practice.

Although it is obvious that *to know* is not necessarily *to do*, nevertheless, that which is done wisely will depend in a large measure on the kind and amount of knowledge one has acquired. In the accumulation of health knowledge, one will need to understand *why* it is beneficial to follow a certain health practice. When one knows why, it is perhaps more likely that a desirable attitude toward certain health practices will be developed. If a person has a sufficient amount of desirable health knowledge developed through valid health concepts, and also has a proper attitude, he or she will be more apt to apply the knowledge in health behavior. Moreover, one should be in a better position to exercise good judgment and make wise decisions in matters pertaining to health if the right kind of knowledge has been obtained.

Health Knowledge

A somewhat frightening lack of knowledge about health was revealed recently in a national health test. In a nationwide sampling, 46 percent of the population had a score of poor; 27 percent, fair; 14 percent, good; and 13 percent, excellent. Among other things, this test indicated that a very small percentage of the population could identify as few as three of the seven early signs of cancer. This is certainly not a very encouraging situation in a nation that is considered to have some of the foremost educational facilities in the world.

Knowledge about health is acquired in a variety of different ways. Some of it is the product of tradition and, as such, oftentimes is nothing more than folklore. Certain popular notions about health-related matters that have long since been dispelled by the scientific community are still held by many people who have not, for some reason or other, benefited from modern health knowledge.

Other kinds of so-called health knowledge are derived from the constant bombardment of the mass media, particularly television and radio. Although some of this information may be valid, we should be alert to the possibility that the primary purpose of many kinds of advertising is to sell a product that proclaims results that are not always likely to be attainable.

Another source of health knowledge is the home, where most health knowledge begins. Parents are our first teachers, and, for better or for worse, what we learn from them, mostly unawares, tends to remain with us. A good home should contribute much to the health knowledge of its children simply by providing good meals and a friendly, well-regulated, pleasant, and recreationally challenging environment. Children from such homes ordinarily do not have to *unlearn* a lot of faulty and unwholesome attitudes when they are in the next great potential source of health knowledge—the schools. It should be borne in mind that many children who grow up in homes in the inner city and some remote parts of the country do not benefit from good home experiences, and thus their first source of health knowledge is in fact the school.

The scope of knowledge that one might obtain about matters related to health is almost endless, and, obviously, it would be impossible to learn all there is to know about it. However, there are certain basic concepts about health that should be developed by individuals at all age levels. Generally speaking, the individual should acquire knowledge pertaining to the direct basic needs of the organism, and, in addition, knowledge regarding the human organism as it functions in its environment. It is well to remember that education is a life-long process, and everyone should attempt to obtain the best health information available from valid sources.

The age-old adage "knowledge is power" is certainly applicable to knowledge about health. When such knowledge is provided under suitable learning conditions, the individual should be empowered to live a fuller and happier life.

Health Attitudes

Any discussion of attitudes requires an identification of the meaning of the term *attitude*. Although it is recognized that different people will attach different meanings to the term, for our purposes, attitude is associated with *feeling*. We hear such expressions as "How do you *feel* about it?" In a sense this implies, "What is your *attitude* toward it?" Therefore, theoretically, at least, attitude could be considered a factor in the determination of action because of this feeling about something. For example, knowledge alone that physical exercise is beneficial will not necessarily lead to regular exercising, but a strong feeling or attitude might be a determining factor that leads one to exercise regularly.

It should be mentioned at this point that, contrary to abundant empirical thought, there is little or no objective evidence to support unequivocally the contention that attitude has a positive direct influence on behavior. One of the difficulties in studying this phenomenon scientifically lies in the questionable validity of instruments used to measure attitudes. Moreover, there is little consistent agreement with regard to the meaning of attitudes. Thus, the position taken here is one of theoretical postulation based on logical assumption.

As far as health attitudes are concerned, they could well be considered a gap that can possibly exist between health knowledge and health practice, and this gap needs to be bridged if effective health behavior is to result from acquiring valid health knowledge. Let us consider, as an example, a person who has acquired some knowledge regarding the degree to which cigarette smoking can be harmful to health. Perhaps one will have some sort of underlying feeling toward such knowledge. He or she may choose to disregard it because friends have also assumed such an attitude. Or it may be felt that the evidence is convincing enough to believe that cigarette smoking is something he or she can get along without. In either case, an attitude has been developed toward the practice of cigarette smoking, and it is likely that one may react according to this feeling. It should also be mentioned that one may not necessarily react in accordance with true feelings because it may be considered fashionable to smoke cigarettes so as not to lose status with friends who do. Whatever way one chooses to react will be tempered at least to an extent by the consequences associated with the knowledge acquired about cigarette smoking.

Obviously, it would be hoped that the accumulation of health knowledge would be accompanied by a positive attitude, and that this attitude would result in desirable action. It is possible that only in terms of such a positive attitude are desirable health practices, and thus a better way of living, likely to result.

Health Practice

It is a well-known fact that all people do not capitalize on the knowledge they have acquired. Perhaps many are apt to act only on impulse; actions of others are influenced to an extent by their friends. However, in a matter as important as one's health, it appears that a reasonable course to follow would be one in which the individual weighs the facts and scientific evidence before acting.

Perhaps we might look at health practices that are desirable and those which are undesirable, or, in other words, those health practices which will result in pleasantness or unpleasantness. If we weigh knowledge in these terms, perhaps we can appreciate better the possible consequence of certain health practices.

Altering behavior is not an easy matter, however, it is hoped that most persons will want to make a positive modification of their own health behavior after acquiring desirable health knowledge and forming favorable attitudes. In the final analysis, children with the help of parent and teacher guidance, will make decisions regarding their own health practices. Perhaps these health practices can be forced, although this notion is impractical if we expect the best learning to take place. Forcing health practices on anyone not only appears impractical but in many cases unwarranted as well.

As far as personal health is concerned, it perhaps becomes a matter of how much risk one is willing to take, and health practices are likely to be based on this factor. By way of illustration, let us refer again to cigarette smoking and health. To my knowledge, it has never been demonstrated scientifically that cigarette smoking is in any way beneficial to the physical health of the human organism. On the contrary, there has been a great deal of medical evidence indicating that smoking can contribute to certain types of serious diseases. Yet in defiance of such evidence, many persons are willing to assume such a dangerous risk. After a person has learned about some aspect of health, he or she is left with an element of choice. It is hoped that a course of healthy action would be chosen so as to minimize risk.

THE MEANING OF HEALTH EDUCATION

My friend the late Dr. Arthur Steinhaus, a notable physiologist, once described *health education* as "any purposeful effort that helps people to change their way of living to add years to life and life to years." Thought of in these terms, health education might well be considered as an area where the specific purpose is teaching children how to live in a healthful and efficient way. In fact, health education could be one of the most important segments of American education because of its concern with teaching how to live well and how to get the most out of life. However, the question arises as to just how our citizenry is going to learn to live in a healthful manner. In the final analysis it will be up to education to prepare children to use the vast amount of health knowledge that has accumulated over the years. Therefore, the job of health education should be to provide desirable health learning experiences for children that will make it possible for them to make the most valid health decisions throughout their lives.

THE MEANING OF FITNESS

Physical fitness has been described in different ways by different people; however, when all of these descriptions are put together, it is likely that they will be characterized more by their similarities than by their differences. For present purposes, physical fitness can be thought of as the level of ability of the human organism to perform various specified physical tasks or, put another way, the fitness to perform tasks requiring muscular effort.

A reasonable question to raise at this point is "why is a reasonably high level of physical fitness desirable in modern times when there are so many effort-saving devices available, that for many people, strenuous activity is really not necessary anymore?" One possible answer to this is that all of us stand at the end of a long line of ancestors, all of whom lived at least long enough to survive in the face of savage beasts and savage men, and were able to work hard. Only the fit survived. As a matter of fact, not very far back in your family tree, you would find people who had to be rugged and extremely active in order to survive. Vigorous action and physical ruggedness constitute our biological heritage. Possibly because of the kind of background that we have, our bodies simply function better when we are active.

There is not complete agreement concerning identification of the components of physical fitness. However, the following information provided by the President's Council on Physical Fitness and Sports considers certain components to be basic:

1. **Muscular Strength.** This refers to the contraction power of muscles. The strength of muscles is usually measured with dynamometers or tensiometers, which record the amount of force particular muscle groups can apply in a single maximum effort. Man's existence and effectiveness depends upon muscles. All movements of the body or any of its parts are impossible without action by muscles attached to the skeleton. Muscles

perform vital functions of the body as well. The heart is a muscle; death occurs when it ceases to contract. Breathing, digestion, and elimination are dependent upon muscular contractions. These vital muscular functions are influenced by exercising the skeletal muscles; the heart beats faster, the blood circulates through the body at a greater rate, breathing comes deep and rapid, and perspiration breaks out on the surface of the skin.

2. **Muscular Endurance.** Muscular endurance is the ability of muscles to perform work. Two variations of muscular endurance are recognized: *isometric,* whereby a maximum static muscular contraction is held, and *isotonic,* whereby the muscles continue to raise and lower a submaximal load, as in weight lifting and performing pushups. In the isometric form, the muscles maintain a fixed length; in the isotonic form, they alternatively shorten and lengthen. Muscular endurance must assume some muscular strength. However, there are distinctions between the two; muscle groups of the same strength may possess different degrees of endurance.

3. **Circulatory-Respiratory Endurance.** Circulatory-respiratory endurance is characterized by moderate contractions of large muscle groups for relatively long periods of time, during which maximum adjustments of the circulatory-respiratory system to the activity are necessary, as in running and swimming. Obviously, strong and enduring muscles are needed. However, by themselves they are not enough; they do not guarantee well-developed circulatory-respiratory functions.

As far as physical fitness is concerned, a major objective of all of us, children and adults, should be in the direction of maintaining a suitable level of physical fitness.

Other Dimensions of Fitness

Up to this point the discussion has been concerned only with physical fitness. Now, let us turn to social fitness, emotional fitness, and intellectual fitness.

Social Fitness

Human beings are social beings. They work together for the benefit of society. They have fought together in time of national emergencies in order to preserve the kind of society they believe in, and they play together.

It was a relatively easy matter to identify certain components of physical fitness such as strength and endurance. However this does not necessarily hold true for the components of social fitness.

Social fitness could be expressed in terms of fulfillment of certain needs. In other words, if certain social needs are being adequately met, we should be in a better position to realize social fitness. Among the needs we must give consideration to are (1) *the need for affection,* which involves acceptance and approval by persons, (2) *the need for belonging,* which involves acceptance and approval of the group, and (3) *the need for self-worth,* which involves one's feelings about his or her own abilities. (The child's social health will be discussed in detail in Chapter 4 — Social Adjustment and Child Health).

Emotional Fitness

Emotion may be described as a response a person makes to a stimulus for which he or she is not prepared or that suggests a possible source of gain or loss. For example, if an individual is confronted with a situation and does not have a satisfactory response, the emotional pattern of fear may result; if a person finds himself or herself in a position where his or her desires are frustrated, the emotional pattern of anger may occur.

This line of thought suggests that emotions might be classified in two different ways — those that are *pleasant* and those that are *unpleasant.* For example, *joy* could be considered a pleasant emotional experience, whereas *fear* would be an unpleasant one. Generally speaking, the pleasantness or unpleasantness of an emotion seems to be determined by its strength or intensity, by the nature of the situation arousing it, and by the way an individual perceives or interprets the situation.

The fact that different individuals will react differently to the same type of situation should be taken into account; for example, something that might anger one person might have a rather passive influence on another individual. In this general connection, it is interesting to note that recently some psychologists and psychiatrists have taken a new look at the emotional pattern of anger. Whereas the old advice was to express one's anger, the recommendation now seems to be to get rid of the thoughts that lead to anger. This is to say that if you avoid anger in the first place you will not need to suppress your anger.

An aspect of controlling the emotions is being able to function effectively and intelligently in an emotionally charged situation. Extremes of emotional upset must be avoided if the individual is to be able to think and act effectively.

It is sometimes helpful to visualize your emotions as being forces within you struggling for power with your mind as to which is to control you, your reason or your emotions. Often our basic emotions are blind and unconcerned with the welfare of other people or sometimes even our own welfare. Emotional maturity has to do with gaining increased mastery over emotions not, of course, eliminating them—so that we may behave as intelligent and civilized human beings rather than as savages or children having temper tantrums. This control is important to emotional fitness. (Chapter 3, Emotional Health of Children, will go into more detail on this subject.)

Intellectual Fitness

The term *intelligence* has been described in many ways. One general description of it is the capacity to learn or understand. Individuals possess varying degrees of intelligence, most people falling within a range of what is called "normal" intelligence. In dealing with this we should give attention to components of intellectual fitness. However, this is a difficult thing to do. Because of the somewhat vague nature of intelligence, it is practically impossible to identify specific components of it. Thus, we need to view intellectual fitness in a somewhat different manner.

For purposes here we will consider intellectual fitness from two different but closely related points of view: first, from a standpoint of intellectual *needs,* and second from a standpoint of how certain things influence intelligence. We might understand better how to contribute to intellectual fitness by improving upon some of these factors.

There appears to be some rather general agreement with regard to the intellectual needs of human beings. Among others, these needs include (1) a need for challenging experiences at the individual's level of ability, (2) a need for intellectually successful and satisfying experiences, (3) a need for the opportunity to solve problems, and (4) a need for the opportunity to participate in creative experiences instead of always having to conform.

Some of those factors which tend to influence intelligence are (1) health and physical condition, (2) emotional disturbance, and (3) certain social and economic factors. When we have a realization of intellectual needs and factors influencing intelligence, perhaps then and only then can we deal satisfactorily with our intellectual pursuits.

Finally, for purpose of this book, the term *children* concerns those in the age range from 5 to 12 years and from grade levels kindergarten to grade six. The following scale shows the approximate ages for children at the various grade levels.

Grade	Age
Kindergarten	5 to 6 years
First Grade	6 to 7 years
Second Grade	7 to 8 years
Third Grade	8 to 9 years
Fourth Grade	9 to 10 years
Fifth Grade	10 to 11 years
Sixth Grade	11 to 12 years

Chapter 2

PHYSICAL HEALTH OF CHILDREN

Physical health of children is concerned with the basic anatomical structure and basic physiological function of the human organism. This means that we should take into account certain physical needs of children. These physical needs are reflected in certain physical characteristics of growing children and this is the major focus of the following discussion.

CHILD HEALTH IN RELATION TO PHYSICAL GROWTH AND DEVELOPMENT

Parents and teachers should be well informed regarding certain principles of child growth and development in order to understand about child health. Although the growth and development of so-called normal children follows a general pattern, it is essential to realize that growth and development is a highly individual matter and that it does not progress at a constant rate. The important thing is not that children grow and develop as others do, but that they grow and develop in their own way, and that they do not stop this process. (For example, a failure to increase in size for a three-month period should be taken as a sign of potential trouble needing medical investigation.) What children's own way of growth and development is depends upon such factors as heredity and particular body build and structure. Therefore, some children of a given age will be slender and some stocky. For them such a condition is healthy. Many parents and teachers have made the mistake of believing that "huskiness" is a criterion for health; and sometimes they have created difficult problems of an emotional kind by attempting to force heavy eating upon children who are naturally slight of build and light eaters.

Parents and teachers should have an intimate knowledge of the physical growth and developmental characteristics of the various age levels of children. The focus of the teacher's attention, although working with a group, needs to remain upon the individual child. Only in this way can the teacher hope to notice the various symptoms associated with abnormalities, including growth and developmental failures.

The following lists of physical characteristics of children have been developed through a documentary analysis of over a score of sources that have appeared in the literature in recent years. It should be understood that these physical characteristics are suggestive of the growth and developmental patterns of the so-called normal child. This implies that if a child does not conform to these characteristics, it should not be interpreted to mean that he or she is seriously deviating from the normal. In other words, it should be recognized that each child progresses at his or her own rate and that there will be overlapping of the characteristics for each of the age levels.

Five-Year-Old Children

1. Boys' height, 42 to 46 inches; weight, 38 to 49 pounds; girls' height, 42 to 46 inches; weight, 36 to 48 pounds.
2. May grow two or three inches and gain from three to six pounds during the year.
3. Girls may be about a year ahead of boys in physiological development.
4. Beginning to have better control of body.
5. The large muscles are better developed than the small muscles that control the fingers and hands.
6. Usually determined whether he or she will be right- or left-handed.
7. Eye and hand coordination is not complete.
8. May have farsighted vision.
9. Vigorous and noisy, but activity appears to have definite direction.
10. Tires easily and needs plenty of rest.

Six-Year-Old Children

1. Boys' height, 44 to 48 inches; weight, 41 to 54 pounds; girls' height, 43 to 48 inches; weight, 40 to 53 pounds.
2. Growth is gradual in weight and height.
3. Good supply of energy.
4. Marked activity urge absorbs him or her in running, jumping, chasing, and dodging games.

5. Muscular control becoming more effective with large objects.
6. There is a noticeable change in the eye-hand behavior.
7. Legs lengthening rapidly.
8. Big muscles crave activity.

Seven-Year-Old Children

1. Boys' height, 46 to 51 inches; weight, 45 to 60 pounds; girls' height, 46 to 50 inches; weight, 44 to 59 pounds.
2. Big muscle activity predominates in interest and value.
3. More improvement in eye-hand coordination.
4. May grow two or three inches and gain three to five pounds in weight during the year.
5. Tires easily and shows fatigue in the afternoon.
6. Has slow reaction time.
7. Heart and lungs are smallest in proportion to body size.
8. General health may be precarious with susceptibility to disease high and resistance low.
9. Endurance is relatively low.
10. Coordination is improving with throwing, and catching becoming more accurate.
11. Whole-body movements are under better control.
12. Small accessory muscles developing.
13. Displays amazing amounts of vitality.

Eight-Year-Old Children

1. Boys' height, 48 to 53 inches; weight, 49 to 70 pounds; girls' height, 48 to 52 inches; weight, 47 to 66 pounds.
2. Interested in games requiring coordination of small muscles.
3. Arms are lengthening and hands are growing larger.
4. Eyes can accommodate more easily.
5. Some develop poor posture.
6. Accidents appear to occur more frequently at this age.
7. Appreciates correct skill performance.

Nine-Year-Old Children

1. Boys' height, 50 to 55 inches; weight, 55 to 74 pounds; girls' height, 50 to 54 inches; weight, 52 to 74 pounds.

2. Increasing strength in arms, hands and fingers.
3. Endurance improving.
4. Needs and enjoys much activity; boys like to shout, wrestle, and tussle with each other.
5. A few girls near puberty.
6. Girls gaining growth maturity up to two years over boys.
7. Girls enjoy active group games, but are usually less noisy and less full of spontaneous energy than boys.
8. Likely to slouch and assume unusual postures.
9. Eyes are much better developed and are able to accommodate to close work with less strain.
10. May tend to overexercise.
11. Sex differences appear in recreational activities.
12. Interested in own body and wants to have questions answered.

Ten-Year-Old Children

1. Boys' height, 52 to 57 inches; weight, 59 to 82 pounds; girls' height, 52 to 57 inches; weight, 57 to 83 pounds.
2. Individuality is well-defined, and insights are more mature.
3. Stability in growth rate and stability of physiological processes.
4. Physically active and likes to rush around and be busy.
5. Before the onset of puberty there is usually a resting period or plateau, during which the boy or girl does not appear to gain in either height or weight.
6. Interested in the development of more skills.
7. Reaction time is improving.
8. Muscular strength does not seem to keep pace with growth.
9. Refining and elaborating skill in the use of small muscles.

Eleven-Year-Old Children

1. Boys' height, 53 to 58 inches; weight, 64 to 91 pounds; girls' height, 53 to 59 inches; weight 64 to 95 pounds.
2. Marked change in muscle system causing awkwardness and habits sometimes distressing to the child.
3. Shows fatigue more easily.
4. Some girls and a few boys suddenly show rapid growth and evidence of the approach of adolescent.

5. On the average, girls may be taller and heavier than boys.
6. Uneven growth of different parts of the body.
7. Rapid growth may result in laziness of the lateral type of child and fatigue and irritability in the linear type.
8. Willing to work hard at acquiring physical skills, and emphasis is on excellence of performance of physical feats.
9. Boys are more active and rough in games than girls.
10. Eye-hand coordination is well developed.
11. Bodily growth is more rapid than heart growth, and lungs are not fully developed.
12. Boys develop greater power in shoulder girdle muscles.

Twelve-Year-Old Children

1. Boys' height, 55 to 61 inches; weight, 70 to 101 pounds; girls' height, 56 to 72 inches; weight 72 to 107 pounds.
2. Becoming more skillful in the use of small muscles.
3. May be relatively little body change in some cases.
4. Ten hours sleep is considered average.
5. Heart rate at rest is between 80 and 90.

It is perhaps appropriate to comment on the ranges of height and weight given here. These heights and weights are what might be called a range within a range, and are computed means or averages within larger ranges. In other words, some children at a given age level could possibly weigh much more or less and be much taller or shorter than the ranges indicate. To illustrate how wide a range can be, one study of a large number of children showed that eleven-year-old girls ranged in weight from 45 to 180 pounds.

TEACHER OBSERVATION OF THE PHYSICAL HEALTH OF CHILDREN

A seven-year-old boy was given several pictures showing some children in good health and some in various states of moderately ill health. Simply on the basis of their general appearance, he was asked to say which children he thought were healthy and which he thought were not feeling well. Without difficulty he distinguished the healthy children, stating happily, "He's healthy," or "She's healthy." Although feelings and health cannot be objectively appraised in this way it does indicate that, generally speaking, the healthy state is usually reflected through signs which are readily observable. These signs include the appearance of alertness and vigor, brightness of the eyes, and keen interest in life. When it is possible to observe the child, the signs of health also include the well-coordinated and confident manner in which he or she moves about, his or her enthusiasm for work and play, and capacity to function reasonably effectively and happily as a group member.

The Daily Health Observation

The teacher's daily observation of his or her class for indications of departures from good health is a key factor in protecting the health of children. In the past, a daily health inspection was a common practice at the elementary school level; however, in more modern times the tendency is to move away from this rather formal approach which relegated "health" to a specified few minutes a day. The health observation should be looked upon as being a continual process which takes place each day and throughout the school day. It should be based upon the teacher's awareness of and sensitivity to matters of child health. The essential features of health observation are: (1) the teacher's constant alertness to matters of health, and (2) the teacher's awareness of the characteristics of normal health at the various age levels and the characteristics of common illnesses of children.

Detection and Referral

The responsibility for continually observing children for evidences of departure from health and the making of suitable referrals does not carry with it the further responsibility of diagnosing specific illnesses. Diagnosis is a matter which rests with medical, psychological, speech and other specialists. However, the more detailed and accurate the teacher's noting of pertinent symptoms, the more valuable the information he or she can provide to those responsible for diagnosis. For example, a comment such as, "George does not seem to feel well today," gives the nurse or physician little specific aid; but a brief account of signs and symptoms exhibited by the child over a period of time that led him or her to believe that George was not feeling well is likely to be much more helpful.

Acute illnesses, such as the onset of measles and appendicitis usually attract attention quickly and offer relatively little difficulty in the way of diagnosis to qualified specialists. On the other hand, the less abrupt departures from health, such as growth failure due to certain diseases or malnutrition, and some behavior disorders in the emotional life of the child, tend to offer greater diagnostic difficulties.

Information that the teacher may provide may be of considerable value in identifying the nature of the child's problem. For example, the teacher may give details about a particular child's increased irritability, reduced vitality, or tendency to withdraw from activities which might not be apparent in an interview or medical examination but which might be important factors in general health appraisal.

The following outline of signs and symptoms is presented merely as a guide to common indications of trouble in regard to child health.

1. **Facial Appearance.** The facial appearance of the child frequently gives an indication of present status. One should be alert to such symptoms as: unusual redness or pallor of the face, inflammation of the eyeballs, and a running nose. Such signs individually or in combination, can be brought on by various diseases, but in any event they are common signs of trouble and should receive attention. Although these symptoms signal the onset of common respiratory illnesses, they are also symptoms of some of the more severe diseases of children.

2. **The Respiratory System.** Respiratory diseases are the principal cause of absenteeism among school children and although they are not usually very severe, in some cases they are quite serious. Colds and other respiratory disturbances are thought to be most contagious in their early stages; that is, within the first two or three days. If children are kept at home when persistent coughing, sneezing, and running noses are observed, infection of large numbers of other children and perhaps the teacher may be avoided. Since many more serious diseases may resemble a simple cold in their early stages, the child should be watched closely for evidence of mounting fever, muscular pain, nausea, and other symptoms. Although there are not at present very effective means of curing colds, children should be taught the importance of wearing proper clothing, eating wisely and getting enough rest in order to keep the frequency and severity of colds to a minimum.

Teachers can easily check mouth breathers to determine whether they are unable to breathe through the nose freely. Inability to breathe easily through the nose is indicative of some form of nasal blockage which should receive medical consideration.

Special note should be made of those individuals who are subject to repeated colds and suitable referrals should be made. Frequent colds may be indicative of a dietary deficiency, some chronic infection, poor dressing habits, or other factors related to a lowered resistance. They may also be related to a disturbed state in the emotional life of the child.

3. **The Eyes.** Certain behavior patterns should give rise to suspicion that the eyes are not functioning properly. For example, a child may hold reading material within a few inches of the face, may squint and make faces as he or she strains to read what is on the chalkboard. One's eyes may be very sensitive to light and he or she may wipe or rub the eyes frequently or close one eye when trying to see. Upon being questioned, the child may complain of blurred vision, headache and dizziness when reading or doing close work, or of not being able to see the ball or other objects when playing games. In appearance, the eyes may be watery and inflamed and the lids swollen and encrusted.

Glasses do not always assure correction of visual defects. When children with glasses show signs of visual difficulty, it is well to bear in mind the possibilities that diagnosis may not have been correct and the glasses do not provide the necessary compensation, or that new difficulties have developed since the previous diagnosis.

Many schools now attempt to provide regular vision testing programs in which all children are screened for visual defects at regular intervals. However, in some cases it may be necessary for the teacher to administer a simple test such as the Snellen test to one or more children.

The teacher can play an important role in encouraging children to wear their glasses, since it sometimes happens that they refuse to wear them for fear of being teased or appearing "different." Skillful teaching can help to make glasses socially acceptable among children.

4. **The Ears.** Partial hearing loss can frequently be identified by certain typical behaviorisms of children. They may strain forward with an intent look when instructions are being given, turn one ear toward the speaker or cup a hand behind the ear. If a child cannot hear his or her own voice well, the speech may become flat and poorly modulated. It sometimes happens that children who appear dull or disinterested in class activities are merely unable to hear clearly what is taking place.

Screening tests should be conducted periodically in order to locate individuals with subnormal hearing. Hearing testing programs are becoming standard practice throughout the country. In localities where programs of this kind are routine, large numbers of cases have been treated which had not been previously suspected. Even though screening is done, the teachers should remain alert to behavior which suggests the possibility of hearing difficulty since infection, injury, and wax accumulation can reduce acuity of hearing rapidly with the result that symptoms may appear suddenly.

5. **The Neck.** Lumps in the neck may be due to mumps which cause a swelling of the salivary glands or to swelling of the lymph nodes just below the ear and behind the jaw. Lumps of either kind should receive the attention of a physician. Swelling of the lymph nodes indicates the presence of infection, perhaps in the gland itself or in some other region of the head, the ear, scalp, or throat.

6. **The Teeth.** Dental screening in schools oftentimes reveals that approximately 80 percent or more of the children are in need of treatment. Although a satisfactory evaluation of dental health requires trained personnel, there are certain gross symptoms which the teacher should recognize. Some of these are: in very bad cases it is possible to see the dark yellow spots of decay at the base and sides of the front teeth; sometimes the foul smell of infection may be perceptible on the child's breath; the gums may be inflamed and sore; the upper and lower sets of teeth may not fit properly together when the mouth is closed; and the very obvious symptoms of toothache. Periodic dental screening should be done by qualified persons, but the teacher must remain alert to gross difficulties.

The teacher can play an important role in helping the child to form a desirable attitude toward having the teeth examined and toward making periodic visits to the dentist.

7. **The Hair and Scalp.** Ringworm is a condition which may be recognized by the forming of nearly bald areas and crustiness of the scalp. It can spread rapidly from child to child.

Pediculi or lice usually appear in regions where living conditions are unhygienic, but they may spread rapidly to anyone who is nearby. The teacher should be able to recognize the pests and become suspicious when the small eggs or nits are discovered clinging to the hair. Frequent itching of the scalp should be investigated for disease or infestation.

8. **Posture.** Poor posture may take several forms such as the head carried too far forward, round shoulders, one shoulder held higher than the other, sway back or forward curvature of the spine, pronated ankles, and flat feet. The poor posture of some children is due to actual deformation of the skeleton and treatment is necessarily a medical matter. Most

cases of poor posture are functional and due to difficulties other than skeletal abnormality.

It should be recognized that although poor posture may be due to bad habits of sitting, standing, and moving, or to the influence of unfortunate fads and styles, it is frequently a symptom of some underlying difficulty. Therefore, it is unwise to require children to begin taking exercises or other corrective measures. For example, it would plainly be unwise to initiate an exercise program for a round shouldered boy if his stance is due to weakness from disease or malnutrition. Similarly, it would be unwise to suggest corrective activities to a child whose head-forward stance represents an attempted compensation for poor vision which actually can only be corrected by glasses. It is known, too, that prolonged emotional upset can be a cause of poor posture, and that improvement must begin with relieving the disturbing situation.

Once underlying causes of poor posture have been removed, the task is to convince the child as to the advantages of good posture and to guide his or her self-analysis so that improvement can take place. Whatever its cause, poor posture may become a habit which is broken only with conscious effort. Therefore, it is plain that children must want good posture if improvement is to take place.

Among very young children, improved use of the feet may result from teaching them to walk and run with the toes pointing forward. Older children can appreciate the principles of body mechanics involved. Of course, severe cases should be referred to a physician for evaluation and possible treatment.

The teacher's guidance can also be of great importance in the matter of selecting proper footwear. Children should be taught to have their feet properly measured and fitted; and they should be taught the hazard to their feet of wearing shoes that are in poor repair. For example, as a heel becomes worn on the inside, additional body weight is thrown upon the inside of the foot and there is an increased tendency towards pronation or forcing the ankle inward and downward.

9. **Speech Difficulties.** Speech defects should be mentioned because of their frequency, oftentimes in combination with hearing loss. The full implication of speech defects cannot be appreciated until they are considered in the light of: (1) their obvious interference with the most essential of our communication media, (2) the impact that they tend to have upon the emotions of the individual who possesses them, both because of the defective communication and because of the typical parental and other

social reactions to them, and (3) the role that emotional upset commonly plays in the formation of speech defects.

Speech difficulties should be approached with caution because inept handling may complicate and aggravate rather than improve them. One specialist on speech once pointed out that most speech problems have their start, not in the mouths of the children but in the mouths of their parents. This statement suggests that emotional problems are intimately involved in the speech situation, and it is likely that therapy in specific cases involves more than practicing saying words or being reminded not to stutter. As a matter of fact, the teacher who has not had specialized training in the area of speech therapy should realize that this difficulty, like a physical or mental disorder, is best left to a specialist.

HELPING CHILDREN LEARN ABOUT THE HUMAN ORGANISM

Child health learning experiences are fundamentally concerned with the basic needs of the body. In the primary grades the areas of emphasis consist of (1) establishing routines and practices conducive to the maintenance of good health; (2) understanding the importance of body cleanliness, including clean hair, nails, skin, and teeth; (3) learning about growth; and (4) caring for teeth, eyes, and ears.

In general, the subject matter for the upper elementary level can be classified under structure and function of the body. The fourth-grade teaching content includes such topics as (1) structure and function of the eyes and ears; (2) identification of the framework and organs of the body; and (3) control of certain communicable diseases. At the fifth-grade level the various systems of the body can be studied. Other health content areas include (1) structure and function of the skeleton, muscles, nerves, and sense organs; and (2) defense against disease. Sixth grade concepts can center around the interdependence of the systems of the body (circulatory, digestive, nervous, respiratory), and glandular functions. Following are some suggested health concepts to be developed. Although formal health teaching takes place in the school, at the same time parents should be aware of the concepts so that they can help children develop them.

Kindergarten

Cleanliness

We wash our hands before we eat.
We wash our hands after going to the toilet.
We take a bath at night.

Growth

We are growing up.
We get weighed and measured to see how much we grow.

Teeth

We brush our teeth after eating.

Grade 1

Cleanliness

We should take a bath and clean our teeth before going to bed.
When we get up in the morning it is important to wash our face and hands.
We should wash our hands before and after eating, after going to the toilet, and after blowing our nose.

Growth

Our body grows during the night as well as during the day.
When weighed and measured regularly we can check on how much we are growing.

Teeth

We can care for our teeth by eating proper foods.
We can care for our teeth by visiting the dentist regularly.
We can care for our teeth by brushing them or rinsing our mouth after meals.

Eyes

Sufficient light on our book helps us protect our eyes.
Sunglasses can help protect our eyes from the strong sunlight.

Ears

Healthy, clean ears are needed for good hearing.
We need to tell a grownup when our ears hurt.

Common Colds

When we have a cold we can try to prevent it from spreading to others.
We use a paper handkerchief and dispose of it.
We cover our nose and mouth when we cough or sneeze.

Elimination

We should go to the toilet before we go to bed at night and when we get up in the morning.

Grade 2

Cleanliness

The morning routine should include washing face and hands, cleaning teeth, cleaning fingernails, brushing hair, and dressing in clean clothes.

Growth

When we walk, stand, and sit correctly we help our bodies grow.
Each boy and girl grows in his or her own way.
Height and weight are measures of growth.

Teeth

We should take care of our baby teeth so that our permanent teeth will be strong and healthy.

Eyes

We can care for our eyes by using a good reading light, keeping our hands away from our eyes, and telling grownups when our eyes hurt, or we are having trouble seeing.
If we wear glasses we need to keep them clean.

Ears

We should try to avoid being hit in the ear.
Loud noises can hurt our ears.

Common Colds

Good health practices, such as eating proper foods, getting enough sleep and rest, and playing in the fresh air and sunshine, help keep us free of colds.

We can help ourselves to keep well by keeping fingers away from our nose and mouth.

Elimination

The practice of going to the toilet regularly can help keep us well.

Grade 3

Cleanliness

We need to assume some responsibility for cleanliness of our bodies.
Baths are important to wash away dirt and germs from our skin.
We use only our own toothbrush, comb and towel to protect our own health and that of others.
We help to keep our hair healthy and attractive by brushing it daily and shampooing it regularly.

Growth

The body is growing constantly.
We each have our own "timetable" for growth.

Teeth

If our teeth are to grow straight and strong, they require good care.
Cavities can form in neglected teeth.
We should use the teeth only for that which they are intended.

Eyes

In caring for our eyes we should hold a book at a comfortable distance away from our eyes for reading.
We should have regular eye examinations and wear glasses when needed.

Ears

We can care for our ears by blowing the nose gently.
It is a good idea to see a doctor when we have an earache.

Illness and Disease

We can build body resistance to common colds by diet, activity, and sleep.

Some illnesses require isolation because they are contagious.

Elimination

Our body rids itself of waste through perspiration, bowel movements, and urination.

Senses

We have five senses which help us to know about and enjoy life.

Skin

A purpose of the skin is to keep our body at the right temperature.
The skin helps prevent germs from entering the body.
The skin carries off some waste through its pores.

Nose

The hairs in our nose help to keep the dirt and germs out of our body.

Lungs

We can get fresh air in our lungs when we play outside.

Heart

When we feel our pulse we feel the pressure of the blood as the heart sends it through the tubes of the body.

Grade 4

Cleanliness

Children should accept some responsibility for their own cleanliness.

Growth

Changes in the body size are an important aspect of physical growth.
We grow at different rates in different ways at different times.

Teeth

We have four kinds of teeth, each useful in a different way.

Cavities may grow until the whole tooth is endangered, unless it receives dental care.

Each tooth has a crown protected by a hard coating of enamel, the neck, and roots.

The pulp in the center of the tooth contains nerves and also blood vessels through which nourishment is brought to the tooth.

Teeth help digest our food through chewing, thus mixing it with saliva.

Eyes

The iris of the eyes regulates the amount of light that enters the eye.

We can help to care for our eyes by sitting a proper distance from a television or movie screen.

We can help our eyes by having the proper amount of light around.

Ears

The special structure of the ear catches sounds and carries them to nerves, which in turn carry messages to the brain.

We can do much to care for our ears by washing them thoroughly but carefully.

It is important to have our ears examined after illness so loss of hearing can be quickly discovered.

Illness and Disease

Disease can be spread by fingers, flies, foods, and air.

Infection involves a fight between the body and the germs that enter it.

When we are immunized we receive medication administered by a doctor as a protection from certain infections.

Digestion and Elimination

Digestion is the process of changing food so that the materials can pass into the blood and be used by the body.

Various parts (teeth, stomach, intestines) of the body aid in the digestion of food.

We can aid digestion by chewing food properly.

Parts of the Body

Some of the parts of the body which carry on its functions are the outer covering of the skin, hair, and nails; the skeletal muscles; and the framework of backbone, ribs, skull, and bones of the legs and arms.

The important organs that carry on specific functions are the brain, heart, liver, lungs, kidneys, bladder, and intestines.

Grade 5

Growth

Our body grows because cells divide to make new cells.

Individual differences in height, weight, and body build among children of the same age are to be expected.

The age at which a person begins to grow tall, the way he or she grows, and the time he or she stops growing, are individual matters.

Mouth and Teeth

The lips, teeth, tongue, taste buds, and salivary glands perform important bodily functions in the sense of taste.

In the mouth food is tasted, ground, and moistened for digestion.

Eyes

The eyeball, iris, pupil, lens, retina, optic nerve, cornea, and tear glands each serve a unique function in helping us to see.

Light, passing through the pupil and lens, throws a picture on the retina, and stimulates the optic nerve, which carries the message to the brain, causing us to see.

Ears

Sounds (vibrations in the air) travel through the ear to the auditory nerve, which reports them to the brain.

The brain tells us the kind of sound and from where it came.

Illness and Disease

The body forms chemicals in the blood stream to fight infection.

The prevention and cure of communicable disease can be based upon what is known about germs, how they spread, and how they are controlled.

Immunization and vaccination are measures used to control disease.

Elimination

The blood, bowels, lungs, kidneys, and skin function to eliminate the body of its waste.

Regularity of elimination by bowels and kidneys indicates that the body is functioning to eliminate waste.

Digestive System

Digestion begins in the mouth, is continued in the stomach, and is completed in the small intestines.
Saliva in the mouth changes the starch in food to sugar.
Proteins begin to dissolve in the stomach.
Digestive juices from the liver that are stored in the gall bladder break fats into tiny drops in the small intestines.
Pancreatice juices and digestive juices from the walls of the small intestines complete the job of digesting carbohydrates, proteins, and fats.
Foods which cannot be digested passes to the large intestines for elimination.

Skin

The skin is composed of three layers, each of which serves a specific purpose.
The epidermis (outer layer of skin) varies in thickness and contains pigments that give the skin color.
The dermis (underlayer of skin) contains blood vessels, nerves, sweat glands, oil glands, and hair and nails, which perform necessary bodily functions.
Below the dermis is a layer of fat cells which cushion the skin.

Nose

The nose is the organ in which the sense of smell begins.
The nose cleans and warms the air before it goes to the lungs.
The parts of the nose which perform important bodily functions are the two nostrils, membranes, hairs, and opening to the Eustachian tube.

Respiratory System

The lungs breathe in oxygen.
Carbon dioxide is the waste from the blood as it comes in contact with the air spaces of the lungs.
The lungs expel carbon dioxide.

Circulatory System

The circulatory system supplies the body with food and oxygen.
The circulatory system aids the body in getting rid of waste.

Structure

The smallest part of our body is the cell.
The body is made up of millions of living cells which require food to grow, to repair themselves, and to produce energy and heat.
The framework of our body consists of the head, neck, trunk, arms, and legs.
The backbone is the supporting center for the framework of the body.
The bones help to give the body its shape.
Some bones support and protect the organs.
The trunk consists of the chest and abdomen, which contain vital organs.
The chest holds and protects the heart and lungs.
The abdomen holds and protects such vital organs as the stomach, intestines, liver, bladder, and kidneys.
Voluntary muscles working in pairs bring about the movements made under our own direction.
Involuntary muscles automatically bring about movements of organs in the trunk, such as work of the heart, lungs, and intestines.

Throat

The parts of the throat which perform important bodily functions are the open chamber, trachea, larynx, esophagus, tonsils and adenoids.
The epiglottis keeps food out of the larynx when we swallow.
Vibrations of the vocal cords in the larynx make us able to speak.
The lips, tongue, palate, and teeth help to formulate speech sounds.

Body Temperature

Our body makes heat by burning the fuel in food we consume.
Vigorous exercise uses more body heat than normal exercise.
When we are well, oral temperature remains at approximately 98.6 degrees and 99.6 degrees by rectum.

Brain and Nerves

Our nerves help us to see, hear, taste, smell, touch, and move.
Through the senses things are stored in the brain and become a part of our memory.

Each part of the brain receives messages from different parts of the body.
One set of nerves carries messages to the brain and another set carries messages away.
Both sets of nerves must be used to make the body move.

Grade 6

Glandular System

The lymph glands constitute one important defense against infection.
Endocrine glands have an important role in regulating growth.
The thyroid gland, located in the neck, affects the body's weight and the nervous system.
Sex glands are important glands used to reproduce the human race.

Growth

Everyone grows in spurts, but not everyone spurts ahead at the same time.
Good diet, proper rest, and exercise help us reach our potential in growth.

Teeth

We can help prevent and control tooth decay.
Healthy gums are important to good health.

Eyes

Light rays enter the pupil of the eye and form a picture on the retina at the back of the eye.
A special nerve from the retina carries the picture to the brain, where it is recognized and interpreted.
Periodic eye examinations by an eye specialist is one means of maintaining good eyesight.

Ears

Sound waves are channeled from the outer ear to the canal leading to the eardrum.
The vibrations of the eardrum set in motion the three small bones in the inner ear.
The inner ear is filled with liquid and lined with tiny threads of nerve cells.

When the liquid of the inner ear is disturbed by the vibrations of the bones, the nerve ends transmit messages to the brain, and hearing takes place.

Illness and Disease

Much research is being conducted today on the causes and cures of diseases.
Tiny organisms called germs and viruses cause many diseases.
White blood cells fight germs and viruses.
The body can build antibodies against certain communicable diseases, whereby making itself immune to the disease.
Diseases can be caused by the lack of certain vitamins in the diet.
Diseases can be caused by harmful bacteria in food, water, milk, and air.
Unsanitary conditions, where harmful bacteria can spread and grow, can contribute to disease.

Digestive System

Digestion changes food so it can be used by the cells of the body.
Digested food is delivered by the blood to the tissues in the form which the cells can use it.

Skin

The skin and mucous membranes act as a protective covering for our body.

Respiratory System

The nose, throat, and lungs are the chief parts of the respiratory system which supply oxygen to all body cells.
Our body needs oxygen from the air to burn the fuel in food to produce energy.

Circulatory System

The circulatory system carries blood to all parts of the body.
The heart is a nonstop pump which helps circulate the blood through the body.
Arteries carry blood away from the heart, and veins carry blood back to the heart.

Skeleton

The spine is made up of many small bones separated from each other by firm, tough cushions.

There are three kinds of bones in the body, each shaped to perform its work efficiently.

Bones are held together by muscles and ligaments.

The muscles move the bones at the joint.

Muscles are arranged in pairs and, when a bone moves, one muscle shortens and the other lengthens.

Control of Body Temperature

Blood circulation helps our body to maintain proper temperature.

If not enough heat is lost in radiation the extra heat is lost by evaporation of perspiration in the skin.

Neuromuscular Coordination

The brain sends nerve impulses to the voluntary muscles which cause them to act.

Voluntary muscles working in pairs and controlled by the brain permit us to move as we wish.

Bodily movements which we cannot control are carried on by involuntary muscles.

Nervous System

The nervous system controls the various actions of the body.

The nervous system enables us to think and act as we wish.

Nerves take messages from the sense organs to the brain.

Information which constantly comes into the brain from the sense organs helps us to think.

Touch and pressure spots on the skin send messages to the brain, which helps us feel the things we touch.

Messages sent to the brain from taste buds on the tongue make us able to taste.

Odors cause cells in the nose to send messages to the brain, and we can smell.

PHYSICAL ACTIVITY AND EXERCISE FOR CHILDREN

When used in connection with the human organism, the term *physical* means a concern for the body and its needs. The term *activity* derives from the word "active," one meaning of which is the requirement of action. Thus, when the two words physical and activity are used together, it implies body action. This is a broad term and could include any voluntary and/or involuntary body movement. When such body movement is practiced for the purpose of developing and maintaining *physical fitness* it is ordinarily referred to as *physical exercise.* We are concerned here with both the broad area of physical activity and the more specific area of physical exercise, and how these factors are concerned with physical fitness of children.

Until relatively recent years we have been aware only of the vast importance of physical activity and exercise to cardiovascular and muscular endurance—and thus improved physical fitness. We now know that regular exercise has important psychological benefits as well, because it can decrease anxiety and increase self-confidence and self-esteem. This is accomplished because exercise helps the body manufacture and release natural drugs that provide what is known as a "high." This occurs because exercise causes morphine-like chemicals (endogenous opioids) to be released by the hormonal system. Also the brain increases its release of beta-endorphins (natural body painkillers) into the blood.

TYPES OF PHYSICAL ACTIVITIES AND EXERCISES FOR CHILDREN

Generally speaking, there are three types of activities that are useful in improving physical fitness: (1) *proprioceptive-facilitative,* (2) *isotonic,* and (3) *isometric.*

Proprioceptive-Facilitative Activities

These activities are those that consist of various refined patterns of movement found in various active games. Important in the performance of these activities are those factors involved in movement: (1) time, (2) force, (3) space, and (4) flow.

Force needs to be applied to set the body or one of its segments in motion and to change its speed and/or direction. Thus, force is concerned with how much strength is required for movement.

In general, there are two factors concerned with *space*. These are the amount of space required to perform a particular movement and the utilization of available space.

All movements involve some degree of rhythm in their performance. Thus, *flow* is the sequence of movement involving rhythmic motion. The above factors are included in most all body movements in various degrees. The degree to which each is used effectively in combination will determine the extent to which the movement is performed with skill. This is a basic essential in the performance of proprioceptive-facilitative activities. In addition, various combinations of the following features are involved in the performance of this type of activity: muscular power, agility, speed, flexibility, balance, and coordination.

Isotonic Activities

These are the type of activities with which most people are familiar. An isotonic activity involves the amount of resistance one can overcome during one application of force through the full range of motion in a given joint or joints. An example of this would be picking up a weight and flexing the elbows while lifting the weight to shoulder height.

Isotonics can improve strength to some extent. They are also very useful for increasing and maintaining full range of motion. Such range of motion should be maintained throughout life if possible, although it can decrease with age and with some musculoskeletal disorders such as arthritis.

Another important feature of isotonic activity is that it can increase circulatory-respiratory endurance in such activities as running and swimming. These activities are usually referred to as *aerobic*.

Isometric Activities

Although isometrics do not provide much in the way of improvement of normal range of motion and endurance, they are most useful in increasing strength and volume of muscles. In isometrics, the muscle is contracted, but the length of the muscle is generally the same during contraction as during relaxation. The contraction is accomplished by keeping two joints rigid while at the same time contracting the muscle(s) between the joints. A maximal amount of force is applied against a fixed resistance during one all-out effort. An example of this is pushing or pulling against an immovable object. Let us say that if one places his or her hands against a wall and pushes with as much force as possible, he or she will have effected the contraction of certain muscles while their length has remained essentially the same.

SCHOOL PHYSICAL ACTIVITY PROGRAMS

Most better-than-average elementary schools try to provide a well-balanced physical education program for children. Just as young children need to learn the basic skills of reading, writing, and mathematics, they should also learn the basic *physical* skills. These include (1) locomotor skills of walking, running, leaping, jumping, hopping, galloping, skipping, and sliding; (2) the auxiliary skills of starting, stopping, dodging, pivoting, landing, and falling; and (3) the skills of propulsion and retrieval involving throwing, striking, kicking, and catching.

For the young child, being able to move effectively and efficiently as possible is directly related to the proficiency with which he or she will be able to perform the various fundamental physical skills. In turn, the success that children have in physical education activities requiring certain motor skills will be dependent upon their proficiency of performance of these skills. Thus, effective and efficient movement is prerequisite to the performance of basic motor skills needed for success in school physical activities. These activities include active games, rhythmic activities, and gymnastic activities. (Parents are advised to explore the extent to which a given school provides for such physical activities for children.)

The extent to which physical activities—particularly through physical education programs—contributes to physical fitness and thus to physical health of children needs to be taken into account. In this regard, sometime ago in what has become a classic report, Dr. G. Lawrence Rarick,[1] Professor Emeritus at the University of California, Berkeley, called attention to some results of research that bear upon physical activity as it relates to physical fitness and development. The following is a summary of some of the highlights of this report.

---

1 Rarick, G. Lawrence, Effects of Physical Activity on the Growth and Development of Children, *The Academy Papers*, No. 8, American Academy of Physical Education, Anaheim, CA, March 27–28, 1974.

1. There is little or no evidence that planned physical activity experiences have an influence on the growth of height of children.
2. There is sufficient information on exercise and muscle growth to provide us with general guidelines in designing physical activity programs if our purpose is to favorably affect general growth and muscular development without overdoing it.
3. One of the most striking effects of vigorous activity during the growing years is its influence upon the child's body composition; that is, the relative amount of lean, fat-free body mass. Some studies have shown that boys included in a vigorous regular physical activity program, as compared to inactive boys, substantially increased their lean body mass at the expense of fat.
4. There is general agreement that moderate stress in the form of vigorous exercise is a positive force in building sturdy bones. However, the difficulty involved in the assessment of the exact influence of physical activity on bone growth makes it almost impossible to evaluate the effect of planned physical activity programs on this aspect of growth.
5. The specific effect of school physical activity programs on the fitness of children shows that little or no solid data collected on a longitudinal basis exists to support the hypothesis made by many physical educators. Studies made on a short-range basis have produced varying and sometimes conflicting results.

In summarizing research findings in this general area, Dr. Rarick suggested that while we know that the stimulus of physical activity is essential to insure the normal physical growth and physiological development of children, we do not know the amount or intensity that is necessary. In addition, its effects most assuredly vary within the individual from one period of development to another and differ widely among individuals. And further, the importance of physical activity in providing for physical fitness of children goes beyond its effect on structural and morphological growth, for its true significance rests on what it does for the child as a functioning, responding being. Finally, without a sound structural organic base, unfortunate limitations are almost certain to be imposed on what might have been a strong, vigorous, and healthy child.

More recently, that is, almost two decades later, I made an extensive review of the literature on this subject and found essentially the same results. One exception has been on the negative side. For example Davis and Isaacs[2] report that extremely long distance running by children can adversely affect long bone growth.

OUT-OF-SCHOOL PHYSICAL ACTIVITY PROGRAMS

Out-of-school programs are provided by various organizations such as boys' and girls' clubs and neighborhood recreation centers. These programs vary in quality depending upon the extent of suitable facilities and qualified personnel available to supervise and conduct them. Parents should investigate these programs thoroughly to make sure they are being conducted in the best interest of children. This is mentioned because some highly competitive sports programs for children place more emphasis on parental pride than on the welfare of children. This should not be interpreted as an indictment against all out-of-school programs because many of them are doing a satisfactory job.

Some families do not rely on any kind of organized out-of-school program, preferring instead to plan their own activities. They make a valid effort to provide activities on their own. This is commendable because it can make for fine family relationships as well as provide for wholesome physical activity for the entire family. There is much truth to the old adage: "The family that plays together stays together."

CURRENT STATUS OF PHYSICAL FITNESS OF CHILDREN

At the present time there is no consistent agreement with regard to the current status of physical fitness of children. One ongoing long-range national study conducted by Dr. Wynn Updyke of Indiana University reports the following findings.

1. The nation's school children have become fatter and less fit during the past decade.
2. If this trend continues it is predicted that these children will be at greater risk for illness as they become adults.
3. This may be a reflection that teachers do not have sufficient time to provide for aerobic fitness as an objective.

---

[2] Davis, Robert G. and Isaacs, Larry D., *Elementary Physical Education*, Winston-Salem, NC, Hunter Books, Inc., 1992

4. Less than one-half (46%) of physical education teachers listed their most important goal as improving physical fitness of students.
5. The others were more interested in improving motor ability (34%), mental health (7%), sports skills (6%), or social skills (6%).
6. The majority of teachers (59%) said the primary objective of physical fitness development is "enhancement of self-esteem" rather than disease prevention, improved appearance, or athletic development.
7. With self-esteem valued so highly, it is suggested that teachers might tend to overemphasize sports and games because they involve more social interaction.

It is interesting to note that not all researchers agree with these findings. For example, Raithel[3] suggests that although many fitness experts and most members of the public believe that American children are unfit, the evidence is inconclusive, and only in terms of body composition are children today known to be less fit than children of 20 years ago.

Another example of the current controversy in regard to the physical fitness of children is found in the comments by Steven N. Blair, M.D., epidemiologist at the Institute for Aerobic Research in Dallas, Texas and Harlen C. Hunter, M.D., President, St. Louis Sports Orthopedic Medicine Clinic.[4]

Dr. Blair, whose Institute has developed the *Fitnessgram,* the first nationally used test with fitness standards established by an expert consensus takes an affirmative stand. He reports that this computer-scored test measures aerobic power, upper body strength, strength and endurance of the abdominal musculature, lower back flexibility and skin folds. Among nearly 40,000 school children, most had acceptable scores, depending upon the age group; 63 to 89 percent passed.

On the contrary, Dr. Hunter maintains that examining children for Little League, it was found that most could not do a good pushup. He has indicated that because of potential risks to health his Clinic has to restrict activities of about 6 percent of children. And further, that the number one reason is hypertension with blood pressure of those under 17 years of age ranging as high as 170/110. In addition, he suggests that if children who want to participate in sports are in such poor condition,

---

[3] Raithel, K. S., Are American Children Really Unfit? *Physicians and Sportsmedicine,* October 1988.

[4] Blair, Steven N. and Hunter, Harlen C., Are American Kids Fit? *HEALTH, A Weekly Journal of Medicine, Science and Society,* September 11, 1990.

those with no interest could be in even worse condition. And finally, about 40 percent of children from ages five to eight show at least one heart-disease risk factor.

HELPING CHILDREN LEARN ABOUT PHYSICAL ACTIVITY AND EXERCISE

Experiences relating to the child's natural urge to play or exercise the body should include indoor and outdoor activities at home and school. Giving the children opportunities to develop the physical skills needed for game participation is the responsibility of both the primary teacher and physical education teacher. The emphasis at the upper elementary level should be on *why* the body needs physical activity and exercise, and *how* it aids growth, development, and bodily functions. Physical education activities appropriate to the growth and developmental level of each child should be an integral part of the health teaching content. Following are some suggested concepts that parents and teachers might try to develop.

Kindergarten

Walking and running is good exercise.
We play games inside on rainy days.
We play out-of-doors after school.

Grade 1

Play helps us grow strong and healthy.
We need to play out-of-doors in the fresh air and sunshine.
Running and jumping help us grow big and strong.

Grade 2

Playing and exercising in the fresh air and sunshine help us grow strong and healthy.
Doing stunts and throwing and catching a ball provide good exercise.
Summer offers many chances for healthful living because there is more time to play out-of-doors.
Playing out-of-doors helps us look well, feel well, and sleep well.

Grade 3

Active play gives us a healthy appetite.
Camping, hiking, and swimming help us build strong and healthy bodies.
When we climb on playground apparatus, we help ourselves to grow bigger and stronger.
Races and relays give us needed exercise.
Exercise helps our bodies to develop different skills.

Grade 4

Daily out-of-door exercise helps to produce strong muscles and a healthy body.
Exercise strengthens the body's defense against disease.
Games and stunts exercise our muscles and help them grow strong.
Bicycling and roller skating are healthful out-of-door activities.

Grade 5

Active out-of-door exercise helps us to sleep, eat, and feel better.
Active play contributes to lung development.
Physical activity and exercise is important to the development of muscles.
Sunshine and fresh air are helpful to all parts of the body.
Exercise stimulates and aids digestion.

Grade 6

There are many ways to get good physical activity and exercise.
Physical activity and exercise helps one to keep fit.
Physical activity and exercise increases the respiration rate.
Physical activity and exercise increases the rate of the heart.
Physical activity and exercise stimulates the heat production of the body.
Physical activity and exercise helps the blood circulate properly.
Physical activity and exercise aids body functions.
Physical activity and exercise conditions the body and adds to its strength, endurance, and agility.
Physical activity and exercise helps improve our self-esteem.

Chapter 3

EMOTIONAL HEALTH OF CHILDREN

At one time or another, most everyone (children, parents, and teachers alike) demonstrates emotional as well as ordinary behavior. Parents and teachers should not necessarily think in terms of always suppressing the emotions of children. On the contrary, the goal should be to help children express their emotions as harmlessly as possible when they do occur so that emotional stability, and thus emotional health will be maintained. If this can be accomplished, problems resulting from harmful emotional behavior can at least be reduced, if not eliminated entirely.

As mentioned in Chapter 1, emotional patterns can be arbitrarily placed into the two broad categories of *pleasant* emotions and *unpleasant* emotions. Pleasant emotional patterns can include such feelings as joy, affection, happiness, and love, while unpleasant emotional patterns can include anger, sorrow, jealousy, fear, and worry—an imaginary form of fear.

The pleasantness or unpleasantness of an emotion seems to be determined by its strength or intensity, by the nature of the situation arousing it, and by the way the child perceives or interprets the situation.

The ancient Greeks identified emotions with certain organs of the body. For example, in general sorrow was expressed from the heart (a broken heart), jealousy was associated with the liver, hate from the gallbladder, and anger with the spleen. In this regard, we sometimes hear the expression "venting the spleen" on someone. This historical reference is made, because in modern times we have taken into account certain conduits between emotions and the body. These are by way of the nervous system and the endocrine system. That part of the nervous system principally concerned with the emotions is the *autonomic* nervous system which controls functions such as the heart beat, blood pressure, and digestion. When there is a stimulus of any of the emotional patterns, these two systems activate. By way of illustration, if the emotional pattern of fear is stimulated the heartbeat accelerates, breathing is more rapid, and the blood pressure is likely to rise. Energy fuel is discharged into the blood from storage in the liver, which causes the blood sugar level to rise. These, along with other bodily functions, serve to prepare a person for coping with the condition that caused the fear.

Dealing with childhood emotions implies that sympathetic guidance should be provided in meeting anxieties, joys, and sorrows, and that help should be given in developing aspirations and security. In order to attempt to reach this objective, we might well consider emotions from a standpoint of the growing child maturing emotionally.

For purposes of this discussion *maturity* is considered as concerned with a state of *readiness* on the part of the organism. The term is most frequently used in connection with age relationships. For example, it may be said that, "Johnny is mature for six years of age." Simply stated, *emotional maturity* is the process of acting one's age.

Generally speaking, emotional maturity will be achieved through a gradual accumulation of mild and pleasant emotions. Emotional *immaturity* indicates that unpleasant emotions have accumulated too rapidly for the child to absorb. One of the important factors in this regard is the process of *adjustment*, which can be described as the process of finding and adopting modes of behavior suitable to the environment or to changes in the environment.

Emotional health is concerned with emotional adjustment. The child's world involves a sequence of experiences that are characterized by the necessity for him or her to adjust. Consequently, it may be said that "normal" behavior is the result of successful adjustment and that abnormal behavior results from unsuccessful adjustment. The degree of adjustment that the child achieves depends upon how adequately he or she is able to satisfy basic needs and fulfill desires within the framework of the environment and the pattern of ways dictated by society.

When a child's needs (basic demands) are not met and his or her desires (wants and wishes) are not satisfied, *frustration* or *conflict* result. Frustration occurs when a need is not met, and conflict results when: (1) choices must be made between nearly equally alternatives, or (2) when basic emotional forces oppose one another. In an emotionally healthy child the degree of frustration is ordinarily in proportion to the intensity of the need or desire. That is, he or she will objectively observe and evaluate the situation to ascertain whether a solution is possible and, if so, what solution would best enable him or her to achieve the fulfillment of needs and desires.

In order to counteract some of the above problems and to be able to pursue a sensible course in helping children become more emotionally mature, there are certain factors concerned with emotional health of children that need to be taken into account. Some of these factors are the subject of the ensuing discussion.

FACTORS CONCERNING EMOTIONAL HEALTH

Some of the factors concerned with emotional health of children that need to be considered are: (1) characteristics of childhood emotionality, (2) emotional arousals and reactions, and (3) factors that influence emotionality.

Characteristics of Childhood Emotionality

Ordinarily the Emotions of Children Are Not Long Lasting

A child's emotions may last for a few minutes and then terminate rather abruptly. The child gets it "out of his system" so-to-speak, by expressing it outwardly. In contrast, some adult emotions may be long and drawn out. As children get older, expressing the emotions by overt action is encumbered by certain social restraints. This is to say that what might be socially acceptable at one age level is not necessarily so at another. This may be a reason for some children developing *moods,* which in a sense are states of emotion drawn out over a period of time and expressed slowly. Typical moods of childhood may be "sulking" due to restraint of anger, being "jumpy" from repressed fear, and becoming "humorous" from controlled joy or happiness.

The Emotions of Children Are Likely to Be Intense

This might be confusing to some adults who do not understand child behavior. That is, they may not be able to see why a child would react rather violently to a situation that to them might appear insignificant.

The Emotions of Children Are Subject to Rapid Change

A child is capable of shifting rapidly from laughing to crying or from anger to joy. Although the reason for this is not definitely known, it might be that there is not as much depth of feeling among children as there is among adults. In addition, it could be due to lack of experience that children have had, as well as their state of intellectual development.

We do know that young children have a short attention span that could cause them to change rapidly from one kind of emotion to another.

The Emotions of Children Can Appear With a High Degree of Frequency

As children get older they manage to develop the ability to adjust to situations that previously would have caused an emotional reaction. This is probably due to the child's acquiring more experience with various kinds of emotional situations. Perhaps a child learns through experience what is socially acceptable and what is socially unacceptable. This is particularly true if the child is reprimanded in some way following a violent emotional reaction. For this reason, the child may try to confront situations in ways that do not involve an emotional response.

Children Differ in Their Emotional Responses

One child confronted with a situation that instills fear may run away from the immediate environment. Another may hide behind the mother. Still another might just stand there and cry. Different reactions of children to emotional situations are probably due to a host of factors. Included among these may be past experiences with a certain kind of emotional situation, willingness of parents and teachers to help children become independent, and family relationships in general.

Strength of Children's Emotions Are Subject to Change

At some age levels certain kinds of emotions may be weak and later become stronger. Conversely, with some children emotions that were strong may tend to decline. For example, small children may be timid among strangers, but later, when they see there is little to fear, the timidity is likely to wane.

Emotional Arousals and Reactions

If we are to understand the emotions of children, we need to take into account those factors of emotional arousal and how children might be expected to react to them. Many different kinds of emotional patterns have been identified. For purposes here, I have arbitrarily selected for discussion the emotional states of fear, worry, anger, jealousy, and joy.

Fear

The term *fear* from the Old English *fir* may have been derived originally from the German word *fahr*, meaning danger or peril. In modern times fear is often thought of in terms of anxiety caused by present impending danger or peril. For example, writing in my series on *Stress in Modern Society*, Whitehead, Shirley and Walker[1] suggest that fear is generally defined as a normal and specific reaction to a genuine threat, which is present at the moment. Anxiety is usually defined as a more generalized reaction to a vague sense of threat in absence of a specific or realistic dangerous object. However, the terms are often used loosely and almost interchangeably. When fearful or anxious, individuals experience unpleasant changes in overt behavior, subjective feelings (including thoughts), and physiological activity.

Similarly, Rathus and Nevid[2] contend that fears differ from anxiety in that the former are negative emotional responses to *specific* situations or objects, such as speaking before a group or receiving an injection, whereas the latter is an emotional state that tends to be prolonged and may be difficult to link to any specific environmental factor. But fears and anxiety are similar in the feelings they arouse: rapid heartbeat, sweating, quivering, heavy breathing, feeling weak or numb in the limbs, dizziness or faintness, muscular tension, the need to eliminate, and a sense of dread. Not all people experience all these signs of fear, but most experience some of them.

Fears are common among children, particularly in early childhood. Examples of such fears are fear of dogs, insects, the dark, and going to school. Childhood fears sometimes appear to be unexplainable and children have marked individual differences in susceptibility to fear. However, there is evidence that children display a definite tendency to learn adult's fears through identification with them or simply by observing them engage in fearful behavior. For example, if during a storm a child observes a parent being fearful, the child is likely to develop a similar fear and fear response pattern. On the other hand, childhood fears are a function of direct contact or experience with frightening events (e.g., if the child were attacked by a dog). Parental warnings,

---

[1] Whitehead, D'Ann, Shirley, Mariela and Walker, C. Eugene, Use of Systematic Desensitization in the Treatment of Children's Fears, In *Stress in Childhood*, Ed. James H. Humphrey, New York, AMS Press, Inc., 1984.

[2] Rathus, Spencer A. and Nevid, Jeffrey S., *Behavior Therapy*, New York, New American Library, 1977.

without the parent necessarily being fearful of such, about certain objects or events (e.g., "watch out for strangers," "stay away from fires") may also lead to developmental fears of children.

Children's fears often tend not to be taken seriously by adults, because some adults generally hold the belief that children's fears "will pass" or that they will "grow out of them." However, it has been found that this may not always be the case, and that without treatment many fears may be maintained through adulthood.

It is possible that sometimes it is not necessarily the arousal itself but rather the way something is presented that determines whether there will be a fear reaction. For example, if a child is trying to perform a stunt and the discussion is in terms of "if you do it that way you will break your neck," it is possible a fear response will occur. This is one of the many reasons for using a positive approach in dealing with children.

A child may react to fear by withdrawing. With very young children, this may be in the form of crying or breath holding. With a child under three years of age (and in some older children as well), the "ostrich" approach may be used; that is the face may be hidden in order to get away from it. As children grow older, these forms of reactions may decrease or cease altogether because of social pressures. For instance, it may be considered "sissy" to cry, especially for boys. The validity of this kind of thinking is, of course, open to question.

Worry

This might be considered an imaginary form of fear and it can be a fear not aroused directly from the child's environment. Worry can be aroused by imagining a situation that could possibly arise; that is, a child could worry about not being able to perform well in a certain activity. Since worries are likely to be caused by imaginary rather than real conditions, they are not likely to be found in abundance among young children. Perhaps the reason for this is that a very young child has not reached the stage of intellectual development at which he or she might imagine certain things that could cause worry. While children will respond to worry in different ways, certain manifestations such as nail biting may be symptomatic of this condition.

An interesting study[3] indicated that children in the 10–11 year age range worry most about the following:

---
[3] The Mini Page, *The Washington Post*, December 25, 1988.

1. AIDS
2. Drugs
3. Dying
4. Grades
5. Homework
6. Moving somewhere else

It is interesting to note that worry about AIDS and drugs may have been prompted mainly by television comments about these subjects, and not necessarily because children have a personal awareness of them. At least this has been demonstrated in some of my interviews with children in this age range.

Anger

This emotional response tends to occur more frequently than that of fear. This is probably because there are more conditions that incite anger. In addition, some children quickly learn that anger may get attention that otherwise would not be forthcoming. It is likely that as children get older they may show more anger responses than fear responses because they soon see that there is not much to fear.

Anger is caused by many factors, one of which is interference with movements that a child may want to execute. This interference can come from others or by the child's own limitations in ability and physical development.

Because of individual differences in children, there is a wide variation in anger responses. These responses are either *impulsive* or *inhibited.* In impulsive responses, the child manifests an overt action either toward another person or an object that caused the anger. For instance, a child who collides with a door might take out the anger by kicking or hitting the door. (This form of child behavior is also sometimes manifested by some "adults.") Inhibited responses are likely to be kept under control, and as children mature emotionally, they acquire more ability to control their anger.

Jealousy

This response usually occurs when a child feels a threat of loss of affection. Many child psychologists believe that jealousy is closely related to anger. Because of this, the child may build up resentment against another person. Jealousy can be devastating in childhood and every effort should be made to avoid it.

Jealousy is concerned with social interaction that involves persons the child likes. These individuals can be parents, teachers, siblings, and peers. There are various ways in which the child may respond. These include: (1) being aggressive toward the one of whom one is jealous or possibly toward others as well, (2) withdrawing from the person whose affections he or she thinks have been lost, and (3) possible development of an "I don't care attitude."

In some cases children will not respond in any of the above ways. They might try to excel over the person of whom they are jealous or they might tend to do things to impress the person whose affections they thought had been lost.

Joy

This pleasant emotion is one for which we strive because it is so important to maintaining emotional stability in children. Causes of joy differ from one age level to another and from one child to another at the same age level. This is to say that what might be joyful for one child might not necessarily be so for another.

Joy is expressed in various ways, but the most common are laughing and smiling, the latter being a restrained form of laughter. Some children respond to joy with a state of relaxation. This is difficult to detect, because it has little or no overt manifestations. Nevertheless, it may be noticed when one compares it with body tension caused by unpleasant emotion.

Factors That Influence Emotionality

If we can consider that a child is emotionally healthy when his or her emotions are properly controlled and he or she is becoming emotionally mature, then emotional health is dependent to a certain extent upon certain factors that influence emotionality in childhood. The following is a description of some of these factors.

Fatigue

Fatigue predisposes children to irritability; consequently, actions are taken to ward it off, such as having rest periods, or, in the case of nursery school, fruit and juice periods. In this particular regard, some studies show that the hungrier a child is, the more prone he or she may be to outbursts of anger. (The conditions of acute and chronic fatigue will be discussed in detail in Chapter 6.)

Inferior Health Status

The same thing holds true here as in the case of fatigue. Temporary poor health, such as colds and the like tend to make children irritable. There are studies that show that there are fewer emotional outbursts among healthy than unhealthy children.

Intelligence

Studies tend to show that, on the average, children of low intelligence have less emotional control than children with higher levels of intelligence. This may be because there may be less frustration if a child is intelligent enough to figure things out. The reverse could also be true, because children with high levels of intelligence are better able to perceive things that would be likely to arouse emotions.

Social Environment

In a social environment where such things as quarreling and unrest exist, a child is predisposed to unpleasant emotional conditions. Likewise, school schedules that are too crowded can cause undue emotional excitation among children.

Family Relationships

There are a variety of conditions concerned with family relationships that can influence childhood emotionality. Among others, these include: (1) parental neglect, (2) overanxious parents, and (3) overprotective parents.

Aspiration Levels

It can make for an emotionally unstable situation if parent expectations are beyond a child's ability. In addition, children who have not been made aware of their own limitations may set goals too high and as a result have too many failures.

All of these factors can have a negative influence on childhood emotionality, and, thus, possibly detract from emotional health. Therefore, efforts should be made as far as possible to eliminate the negative aspects of these factors. Those that cannot be completely eliminated should at least be kept under control.

EMOTIONAL NEEDS OF CHILDREN

In order to understand better the emotional health of children we should be aware of their emotional needs. Among these basic emotional needs are: (1) the need for a sense of security and trust, (2) the need for self-identity and self-respect, (3) the need for success, achievement, and recognition, and (4) the need for independence.

Emotional maturity could be expressed in terms of the fulfillment of these general emotional needs. More specific emotional needs can be reflected in the developmental characteristics of growing children. A number of such emotional characteristics are identified in the following lists at the different age levels.

Five-Year-Old Children

1. Seldom shows jealousy toward younger siblings.
2. Usually sees only one way to do a thing.
3. Usually sees only one answer to a question.
4. Inclined not to change plans in the middle of an activity, but would rather begin over.
5. Some may fear being deprived of mother.
6. Some definite personality traits evidenced.
7. Is learning to get along better, but still may resort to quarreling and fighting.
8. Likes to be trusted with errands.
9. Enjoys performing simple tasks.
10. Wants to please and do what is expected of him or her.
11. Is beginning to sense right and wrong in terms of specific situations.

Six-Year-Old Children

1. Restless and may have difficulty in making decisions.
2. Emotional pattern of anger may be difficult to control at times.
3. Behavior patterns may often be explosive and unpredictable.
4. Jealousy toward siblings at times; at other times takes pride in siblings.
5. Greatly excited by anything new.
6. Behavior susceptible to shifts in direction, inwardly motivated and outwardly stimulated.
7. May be self-assertive and dramatic.

Seven-Year-Old Children

1. Curiosity and creative desires may condition responses.
2. May be difficult to take criticism from adults.
3. Wants to be more independent.
4. Reaching for new experiences and trying to relate himself or herself to enlarged world.
5. Overanxious to reach goals set by parents and teachers.
6. Critical of self and sensitive to failure.
7. Anger is more controlled.
8. Becoming less impulsive and boisterous in actions than at six.

Eight-Year-Old Children

1. Dislikes taking much criticism from adults.
2. Can give and take criticism in his or her own group.
3. May develop enemies.
4. Does not like to be treated as a child.
5. Has a marked sense of humor.
6. First impulse is to blame others.
7. Becoming more realistic and wants to find out for himself or herself.

Nine-Year-Old Children

1. May sometimes be outspoken and critical of the adults they know, although they have a genuine fondness for them.
2. Respond best to adults who treat them as individuals and approach them in an adult way.
3. Likes recognition for doing a task and responds well to deserved praise.
4. Likely to be backward about public recognition, but likes private praise.
5. Developing loyalty and sympathy to others.
6. Does not mind criticism or punishment if it is fair but is indignant if it is unfair.
7. Disdainful of danger to and safety of self, which may be a result of increasing interest in activities involving challenge.

Ten-Year-Old Children

1. Increasing tendency to rebel against adult domination.
2. Capable of loyalties and hero worship, and can inspire it in schoolmates.
3. Can be readily inspired to group loyalties in club organization.
4. Likes the sense of solidarity that comes from keeping a group secret as a member of a group.
5. Each sex has increasing tendency to show lack of sympathy and understanding with the other.
6. Boys' and girls' behavior and interests becoming increasingly different.

Eleven-Year-Old Children

1. If unskilled in group games and game skills, may tend to withdraw.
2. Boys may be concerned if they feel they are underdeveloped.
3. May appear to be indifferent and uncooperative.
4. Moods change quickly.
5. Wants to grow up, but may be afraid to leave childhood security behind.
6. Increase in self-direction and in a serious attitude toward work.
7. Need for approval to feel secure.
8. Beginning to have a fully developed idea of own importance.

Twelve-Year-Old Children

1. Beginning to develop a truer picture of morality.
2. Clearer understanding of real causal relations.
3. The process of sexual maturation involves structure and physiological changes with possible perplexing and disturbing emotional problems.
4. Personal appearance may become a source of great conflict, and learning to appreciate good grooming or the reverse may be prevalent.
5. May be very easily hurt when criticized or made the scapegoat.
6. Maladjustment may occur when there is not a harmonious relationship between child and adults.

These characteristics reflect some of the emotional needs of children at the different age levels; and should be taken into account in both the home and school environments if we expect to meet with success in our efforts to help children develop emotionally.

SOME GUIDELINES FOR THE EMOTIONAL HEALTH OF CHILDREN

It is imperative to set forth some guidelines for the emotional health of children. The reason for this is to assure, at least to some extent, that our efforts in attaining optimum emotional health will be based on a scientific approach. These guidelines might well be taken in the form of *concepts of emotional development.* This approach enables us to give serious consideration to what is known about how children grow and develop. The following list of concepts is submitted with this general idea in mind.

1. **An emotional response may be brought about by a goal's being furthered or thwarted.** The teacher should make a very serious effort to assure successful experiences for every child. This can be accomplished in part by attempting to provide for individual differences within given school experiences. The school setting should be such that each child derives a feeling of personal worth through making some sort of positive contribution.

2. **Self-realization experiences should be constructive.** The opportunity for creative experiences that afford the child a chance for self-realization should be inherent in school. Teachers might well consider planning with children to see that all school activities are meeting their needs and as a result, involve constructive experiences.

3. **Emotional responses increase as the development of the child brings greater awareness and the ability to remember the past and to anticipate the future.** In both the home and school setting the parent and the teacher can remind the children of their past pleasant emotional responses with words of praise. This could encourage children to repeat such responses later in similar situations and thus provide a better learning situation.

4. **As the child develops, the emotional reactions tend to become less violent and more discriminating.** A well-planned program of school experiences and wholesome home activities should be such that it provides for release of aggression in a socially acceptable manner.

5. **Emotional reactions tend to increase beyond normal expectancy toward the constructive or destructive reactions on the balance of furthering or hindering experience of the child.** For some children the confidence they need to be able to face the problems of life may come through physical

expression. Therefore, experiences such as a good physical education program in the schools have tremendous potential to help contribute toward a solid base of total development.

6. **Depending on certain factors, a child's own feelings may be accepted or rejected by the individual.** Children's school experiences should make them feel good and have confidence in themselves. Satisfactory self-concept is closely related to body control; physical-activity-oriented experiences might be considered as one of the best ways of contributing to it. Therefore, it is important to consider those kinds of experiences for children that will provide them with the opportunity for a certain degree of freedom of movement.

OPPORTUNITIES FOR IMPROVING EMOTIONAL HEALTH IN THE SCHOOL ENVIRONMENT

The school has the potential to provide for emotional stability. The extent to which this actually occurs is dependent primarily on the kind of emotional climate provided by the teacher. For this reason, it appears pertinent to examine some of the potential opportunities that exist for the improvement of emotional health in the school setting. It should be borne in mind that these opportunities will not accrue automatically, but that teachers need to work constantly to try to make such conditions a reality.

1. **Release of aggression in a socially acceptable manner.** This appears to be an outstanding way in which school activities such as physical education can help to make children more secure and emotionally stable. For example, kicking a ball in a game of kickball, batting a softball, or engaging in a combative stunt can afford a socially acceptable way of releasing aggression.

2. **Inhibition of direct response of unpleasant emotions.** This statement does not necessarily mean that feelings concerned with such unpleasant emotions as fear and anger should be completely restrained. On the contrary, the interpretation should be that such feelings can take place less frequently in a wholesome school environment. This means that opportunities should be provided to relieve tension rather than aggravate it.

3. **Promotion of pleasant emotions.** Perhaps there is too much concern with suppressing unpleasant emotions and not enough attention given to promoting the pleasant ones. This means that the school should provide

a range of activities by which all children can succeed. Thus, all children, regardless of ability, should be afforded the opportunity for success at least some of the time.

4. **Recognition of one's abilities and limitations.** It has already been mentioned that a wide range of activities should provide an opportunity for success for all. This should make it easier in the school setting to provide for individual differences of children so that all of them can progress within the limits of their own skill and ability.

5. **Understanding about the ability and achievement of others.** In the school experience emphasis can be placed upon achievements of the group, along with the function of each individual in the group. Team play and group effort is important in most school situations.

6. **Being able to make a mistake without being ostracized.** In the school setting this requires that the teacher serve as a catalyst who helps children understand the idea of trial and error. Emphasis can be placed on *trying* and on the fact that one can learn not only from his or her own mistakes but also from the mistakes of others.

This discussion has included just a few examples of the numerous opportunities to help provide for improving emotional health in the school environment. The resourceful and creative teacher should be able to expand this list manyfold.

TEACHER OBSERVATION OF THE EMOTIONAL HEALTH OF CHILDREN

It is difficult to specify a list of behavior traits which always signal poor emotional health because virtually all such traits are observed in the most normal of persons at one time or another. For example, daydreaming is commonly indicated as a symptom of "withdrawn" behavior; and yet we know that all normal children daydream, and we know that various factors such as boredom and emotional stress commonly lead to increased daydreaming. I have expressed my own sentiments in one of my most recent books[4] by stating that "More often than not children are reprimanded in school for 'daydreaming.' This is unfortunate because when one considers a day dream to be 'a pleasant reverie of wish fulfillment,' it could be a form of meditation whereby the child

---

4 Humphrey, James H., *Stress Management for Elementary Schools*, Springfield, IL, Charles C Thomas Publisher, 1993.

extricates himself or herself from the cares and worries of the school day."

Consequently, when evaluating behavior for evidence of poor emotional health, it is necessary to think in terms of *persisting* and *extreme* traits. Thus, habitual daydreaming may suggest a tendency to withdraw from reality. Similarly, habitual defiance of adult authority, cruelty, or extreme excitability would suggest a need for careful investigation by specialists so that the cause might be discovered. Although isolated episodes of these things might deserve noting, they would not in themselves necessarily be symptoms of behavior disorders.

The following list includes some behaviorisms which are sometimes associated with disturbance at the psychological level. *Individual cases must, of course, be reckoned with in terms of persistence and severity of the symptoms.*

Withdrawnness, shyness, seclusiveness, timidity
Daydreaming
Fearfulness, strong anxiety
Tenseness, excitability and lack of emotional control
Extreme desire to please
Lack of self-confidence, an "I can't" attitude
Inability to assume responsibility for own errors
Unhappiness, feelings of depression
Suspiciousness
Avoidance of need to adjust to others
Inability to adjust to the group, especially at play
Nail-biting, habit tics, finger or lip-sucking
Hostile and aggressive behavior
Destructiveness
Cruelty
Temper tantrums, Irresponsibility
Showing off and other attention-getting activities
Lying, cheating, stealing
Lack of self-control
Preoccupation with sex
Failure to make progress which is in keeping with physical and mental capacity

Because so many of the emotional conditions among adults had their beginning in childhood, it is extremely important that teachers be ever alert to the emotional deviations among children that may be the insidious beginning of emotional ill health which reaches its climax in adult life.

HELPING CHILDREN LEARN ABOUT EMOTIONAL HEALTH

All teaching situations, whether during lessons devoted to health or not, should be such that the child has the opportunity to grow and develop to a high degree of emotional stability. The following concepts might serve as examples of some of the more significant aspects of emotional health.

Kindergarten

We feel more comfortable when we know what is expected of us.
We can work alone.
Everyone is different.
Everyone makes mistakes.
We talk things over with our parents.

Grade 1

Getting ready and being on time at home and at school are two ways to show we are growing up.
When we amuse ourselves and do some things on our own we show people we are growing up.
If we have fears we should talk about them with our parents.
Differences help to make life more interesting.
If we make mistakes we should learn from these mistakes.
It is better to control our feelings and to find other things to do than to quarrel.

Grade 2

We are responsible for what we do.
When we make others happy we make ourselves happy.
As we grow up, we can think of different ways to do things and different things to do.
It helps when we are considerate of the mistakes of others.

When something goes wrong it helps to try to be cheerful and to find something else to do.

Grade 3

We can each do some things well.
It helps us to know what we can do well.
A sense of humor can often make things better for everyone.
When we plan we make things easier for ourselves and others.
It helps to make the best of a situation we cannot change.

Grade 4

A happy family is one in which each member makes a contribution to the happiness of others.
For happy group living one needs to respect the rights and wishes of others.
Thoughtfulness and consideration make for pleasant relationships with others.
Everyone should have confidence in his or her own ability and be willing to try new experiences.
Almost everyone has unpleasant feelings sometimes.
Ways of handling disturbed feelings is something each of us must learn.

Grade 5

A mature person assumes responsibility for his or her own health, safety, and behavior, as well as the health and safety of younger children.
Being able to plan ahead is a sign of increasing maturity.
We need to meet our problems and to solve them without anger, jealousy, or unhappiness to ourselves or others.
A responsible person completes a task when it needs to be done.
A responsible person knows when to ask for help.
Control of emotions is important for maintenance of proper bodily function.

Grade 6

We grow physically, socially, intellectually, and emotionally.
Growing up emotionally means growing up in an understanding of our own feelings, and in the ways we handle our feelings.

Control of emotions helps us accomplish our tasks and enjoy life.

Mature people understand and respect their families, friends, and other people.

An awareness of and respect for the feelings of others is evidence of growing up emotionally.

Self-confidence is gained by setting worthwhile goals for ourselves and working toward their attainment.

Talking over our problems and feelings with someone we trust helps to get rid of the problem.

Chapter 4

SOCIAL HEALTH OF CHILDREN

To the best of my knowledge[1] the term *social* was first associated with health when the American *Social* Hygiene Association was formed in 1913. A major function of this organization was to exert an effort to try to stop the spread of venereal diseases. These diseases were considered as "social diseases" at that time; hence, the introduction of the word "social" to the field of health. In the present context *social health* is concerned with the importance of social adjustment. Social maladjustment in children can seriously impact on their emotional health possibly predisposing them to some forms of physical anomaly.

In consideration of social health we need to think in terms of social development. Social development is so comprehensive that it has been described in a number of ways as follows: (1) the pattern of change through the years exhibited by the individual as a result of his or her interaction with such forces as people, social institutions, social customs, and social organizations; (2) the entire series of progressive changes from birth to death in social behavior, feelings, attitudes, values, etc. that are normal for the individual of a species; (3) the state of any moment of an individual's social or socially significant reaction, evaluated in accordance with what is regarded as normal for that culture; (4) the growth of the culture of the group in the direction of the more complete satisfaction of the needs of its members.[2]

SOCIAL NEEDS OF CHILDREN

The importance of social needs is brought more clearly into focus when we consider that most of what human beings do they do together. Social maturity, and thus social health—so important to social development—

---

[1] Humphrey, James H., The New Sex Education, In *Selected Works of James H. Humphrey*, Ed. Joy N. Humphrey, New York, AMS Press, Inc., 1987.

[2] Good, Carter V., *Dictionary of Education*, New York, McGraw-Hill, 1959, p. 168.

might well be expressed in terms of the fulfillment of certain needs. In other words, if certain social needs are being met, the child should be in a better position to realize social health. Among other needs, we must give consideration to (1) the need for *affection* which involves acceptance and approval by persons; (2) the need for *belonging* which involves acceptance and approval of the group; and (3) the need for *mutuality* which involves cooperation, mutual helpfulness, and group loyalty.

When it comes to evaluating social outcomes, we do not have the same kinds of objective instruments that are available in computing accurately the physical attributes of children. In some cases (and primarily for diagnostic purposes) in dealing with children some school systems have successfully used some of the acceptable *sociometric* techniques. However, at best the social aspect is difficult to appraise objectively because of its somewhat vague nature. (These techniques will be discussed later in the chapter.)

In addition to the general social needs previously mentioned, specific needs are reflected in the developmental traits and characteristics of growing children. Many such characteristics are identified in the following lists at the different age levels.

Five-Year-Old Children

1. Interested in neighborhood games that involve any number of children.
2. Plays various games to test his or her skill.
3. Enjoys other children and likes to be with them.
4. Interests are largely self-centered.
5. Seems to get along best in small groups.
6. Shows an interest in home activities.
7. Imitates at play.
8. Gets along well in taking turns.
9. Respects the belongings of other people.

Six-Year-Old Children

1. Self-centered and has need for praise.
2. Likes to be first.
3. Indifferent to sex distinction.

4. Enjoys group play when groups tend to be small.
5. Likes parties but behavior may not always be decorous.
6. The majority enjoy school association and have a desire to learn.
7. Interested in conduct of friends.
8. Boys like to fight and wrestle with peers to prove masculinity.
9. Shows an interest in group approval.

Seven-Year-Old Children

1. Wants recognition for individual achievements.
2. Sex differences are not of great importance.
3. Not always a good loser.
4. Conversation often centers around family.
5. Learning to stand up for own rights.
6. Interested in friends and is not influenced by their social or economic status.
7. May have nervous habits such as nail biting, tongue sucking, scratching, or pulling at ear.
8. Attaining orientation in time.
9. Gets greater enjoyment from group play.
10. Shows greater signs of cooperative efforts.

Eight-Year-Old Children

1. Girls are careful of their clothes, but boys are not.
2. Leaves many things uncompleted.
3. Has special friends.
4. Has longer periods of peaceful play.
5. Does not like playing alone.
6. Enjoys dramatizing.
7. Starts collections.
8. Enjoys school and dislikes staying home.
9. Likes variety.
10. Recognition of property rights is well established.
11. Responds well to group activity.
12. Interest will focus on friends of own sex.
13. Beginning of the desire to become a member of a club.

Nine-Year-Old Children

1. Wants to be like others, talk like others, and look like them.
2. Girls are becoming more interested in their clothes.
3. Is generally a conformist and may be afraid of that which is different.
4. Able to be on his or her own.
5. Able to be fairly responsible and dependable.
6. Some firm and loyal friendships may develop.
7. Increasing development of qualities of leadership and followership.
8. Increasing interest in activities involving challenges and adventure.
9. Increasing participation in varied and organized group activities.

Ten-Year-Old Children

1. Begins to recognize the fallibility of adults.
2. Moving more into a peer-centered society.
3. Both boys and girls are amazingly self-dependent.
4. Self-reliance has grown and at the same time intensified group feelings are required.
5. Divergence between the two sexes is widening.
6. Great team loyalties are developing.
7. Beginning to identify with one's social contemporaries of the same sex.
8. Relatively easy to appeal to his or her reason.
9. On the whole, has a fairly critical sense of justice.
10. Boys show their friendship with other boys by wrestling and jostling with each other, while girls may walk around with arms around each other as friends.
11. Interest in people, in the community, and in affairs of the world is keen.
12. Interested in social problems in an elementary way and likes to take part in discussions.

Eleven-Year-Old Children

1. Internal guiding standards have been set up, and although guided by what is done by other children, he or she will modify behavior in line with those standards already set up.

2. Does a number of socially acceptable things, not because they are right *or* wrong.
3. Although obsessed by standards of peers, he or she is anxious for social approval of adults.
4. Need for social companionship of children their own age.
5. Liking for organized games becoming more prominent.
6. Girls are likely to be self-conscious in the presence of boys and are usually much more mature than boys.
7. Team spirit is very strong.
8. Boys' and girls' interests are not always the same, and there may be some antagonism between the sexes.
9. Often engages in silly behavior, such as giggling and clowning.
10. Girls are more interested in social appearance than are boys.

Twelve-Year-Old Children

1. Increasing identification of self with other children of his or her own sex.
2. Increasing recognition of fallibility of adults.
3. May see himself or herself as a child and adults as adults.
4. Getting ready to make the difficult transition to adolescence.
5. Pressure is being placed on individual at this level to begin to assume adult responsibilities.

GUIDELINES FOR SOCIAL HEALTH

When we have some basis for the social behavior of children as they grow and develop we are then in a better position to select and conduct experiences that are likely to be compatible with their social health. The following list of concepts of social development are submitted with this general idea in mind.

1. **Interpersonal relationships are based on social needs.** All children should be given an equal opportunity in participation. Moreover, the teacher should impress upon children their importance to the group. This can be done in connection with most group efforts, which is so essential to successful participation.

2. **A child can develop his or her self-concept through undertaking roles.** A child is more likely to be aware of his or her particular abilities if given the opportunity to play different roles in school situations. Rotation of

such responsibilities as group leaders and committee assignments tend to provide opportunity for self-expression of children through role playing.

3. **There are various degrees of interaction between individuals and groups.** School experiences should provide for settings for the child to develop interpersonal interaction. The teacher has the opportunity to observe children in various situations. Consequently, the teacher is in a good position to guide integrative experiences by helping children to see the importance of satisfactory relationships in certain group situations.

4. **Choosing and being chosen—an expression of a basic need—is the foundation of interpersonal relationships.** As often as possible, children should be given the opportunity for choosing teammates, partners, and the like. However, great caution should be taken by the teacher to see that this is carried out in an equitable way. The teacher should devise ways of choice so that certain children are not always selected last or left out entirely.

5. **Language is a basic means and essential accompaniment of socialization.** Children can be taught the language of the body through using the names of its parts. This is an important dimension in the development of body awareness. School experiences should be such that there is opportunity for oral expression among and between children. For example, in the evaluation phase of a lesson, children have a fine opportunity for meaningful oral expression if the evaluation is skillfully guided by the teacher.

6. **Learning to play roles is a process of social development.** A child should be given the opportunity to play as many roles as possible in his or her school experiences. This could be involved in the organization of class activities.

7. **Integrative interaction tends to promote social development.** Spontaneity can be considered as one of the desired outcomes of integrative experiences, which means the opportunity for actions and feelings expressed by the child as he or she really is.

8. **Resistance to domination is an active attempt to maintain one's integrity.** The teacher might well consider child resistance as a possible indicator of teacher domination. If this occurs, the teacher might look into his or her actions, which may be dominating the teaching-learning situation. Child resistance should be interpreted as a sign of a healthful personality, and a wise teacher will likely be able to direct the energy into constructive channels to promote social development.

9. **Interpersonal interaction between children is a basis for choice.** If children are left out by other children, this symptom should be studied with care to see if this is an indication of poor interpersonal relationships with other children. Very interesting aspects of interpersonal relationships can be observed by the wise teacher. Children may realize the value of a child to a specific activity and accept such a child accordingly. On the other hand, they may be likely to accept their friends regardless of their ability.

10. **A child, in and as a result of belonging to a group develops differently than he or she can as an individual alone.** Many school activities provide for an outstanding opportunity for children to engage actively in a variety of group experiences. Merely being a member of a group can be a most rewarding experience for a child. If properly conducted, many group activities should provide an optimal situation for desirable social development.

IMPLICATIONS OF RESEARCH IN SOCIAL BEHAVIOR OF CHILDREN

There has been an appreciable amount of research regarding social behavior of children. This being the case, we should perhaps consider some of this research so that we can draw some implications for certain school experiences. This is to say that in utilizing such findings, we will be better able to conduct school experiences that will be more likely to result in improved social health. A report by the National Institute of Education has provided some information that should be useful for this purpose.

The purpose of the report was to provide teachers with a summary of psychological research concerned with the social behavior of young children. In submitting the report, it was noted that caution should prevail with reference to basic research and practical application. In this regard, the following suggestions are submitted.

1. What seems "true" at one point in time often becomes "false" when new information becomes available or when new theories change the interpretation of old findings.
2. Substantial problems arise in any attempt to formulate practical suggestions for professionals in one discipline based on research from another discipline.
3. Throughout the report, recommendations for teachers have been

derived from logical extensions of experimental findings and classroom adaptations of experimental procedures.
4. Some of the proposed procedures may prove unworkable in the classroom, even though they may make sense from a psychological perspective.
5. When evaluating potential applications of psychological findings it is important to remember that psychological research is usually designed to derive probability statements about the behavior of groups of people.
6. Individual teachers may work better with a procedure that is, on the average, less effective.

The following list of generalizations have been derived from the findings. In considering these generalizations the above cautions should be kept in mind. Moreover, each individual teacher will no doubt be able to draw his or her own implications and make practical applications that apply to particular situations.

1. **Reasoning with an emphasis on consequences for other people is associated with the development of a humanistic concern for others.** Teachers might consider encouragement of social behavior in school experiences by discussing the implications of children's and teachers' actions for the feelings of others; poor performers should be encouraged rather than ridiculed.

2. **Children tend to show empathy toward individuals similar to themselves.** In school experiences it is important to emphasize the likenesses of people; while all children may differ in one or more characteristics, they still are more alike than they are different.

3. **Children may learn techniques for positive social interaction by observing children who are behaving cooperatively.** In certain activities, cooperation of each individual is very important to the success of the group; the teacher can suggest ways children can cooperate and reinforce children when these suggestions are followed.

4. **The more frequently children voluntarily practice social skills, the more likely they are to use these skills in less structured situations.** In some school situations children can be assigned certain responsibilities that require the practice of social skills.

5. **Children are likely to use behaviors for which they have been reinforced.** The teacher can focus his or her attention on children who are cooperating, sharing, and helping the teacher and other children in the various school situations.

6. **Children are likely to imitate behaviors for which they see other children being reinforced.** The teacher can compliment those children who are saying cooperative, helpful things to each other. At the same time, the teacher should consider simultaneously ignoring negative social interactions of children.

7. **Children are likely to help and share when they have seen someone else do it, particularly if they know and like the model.** The teacher can take the lead by providing examples of sharing, helping, and cooperating.

8. **Ignored behavior may increase at first, but eventually it is likely to decrease if the child does not receive reinforcement from other sources.** The teacher may wish to pointedly ignore misbehavior whenever possible by turning away from the misbehaving child and attending to a child who is behaving appropriately. Obviously, all misbehavior cannot be ignored because in some instances such misbehavior might be concerned with safety factors. Thus, it is sometimes appropriate for the teacher to act expediently.

9. **Consistent, immediate punishment may tend to discourage the behavior it follows.** When it is necessary, the teacher might consider choosing mild punishment related to the activity, which can follow misbehavior immediately. For example, if a child is misusing a piece of material, it can be removed, at least temporarily.

10. **Reasoning can increase children's awareness of the needs of others, and it (reasoning) is a form of attention that should be limited to occasions when children are behaving appropriately.** In many teaching-learning situations there is a need for certain rules and regulations. It might be well to discuss the reasoning behind rules when children are following the rules and *not* when the rules are disobeyed. However, this does not necessarily preclude a negative approach if a given situation warrants it.

In closing this discussion, it should be reiterated that each individual reader will no doubt be able to draw his or her own implications and make practical applications that apply to particular school situations.

EVALUATING CONTRIBUTIONS OF SCHOOL EXPERIENCES TO SOCIAL HEALTH

In the past, most of what has been done in evaluating social growth in school has been of a subjective nature. The process of "observation" has been considered satisfactory, because it has been felt that for the most part we can merely watch children to see the kinds of relationships that exist between them.

Some educators have approached this problem from a more scientific standpoint and have used certain *sociometric techniques* with varying degrees of success. Included among such techniques are (1) sociograms, (2) sociographs, and (3) social distance scales.

Sociograms

In this technique, a child is usually asked to name in order of preference those persons liked best in a group. A child may be asked to name those he or she would like to be with or play with most. After the choices are made, the results are plotted on a sociogram.

If two children choose each other, they are known as "mutual choices of pairs." Those not selected by anyone in the group and who do not choose anyone are called "isolates." "Islands" is the name given to pairs or small groups of mutual choices not selected by any of the large group. While the sociogram is a worthwhile device for identifying certain aspects of interpersonal relationships, it is a time-consuming procedure and for this reason is not one of the more popular methods used by teachers.

Sociographs

The sociograph is a more expedient and practical way of tabulating and interpreting data. Instead of plotting as in a sociogram, choices are recorded in tabular form opposite the names of children. This readily shows the number of rejections, mutual choices, choices received, and choices given.

Social Distance Scales

This sociometric technique has been used in research in social psychology for well over fifty years. In this procedure, each member of a group is asked to check the other members according to certain degrees of social intimacy such as:

1. Would like to have him/her as one of my best friends.
2. Would like to have him/her in my group, but not as a close friend.

3. Would like to be with him/her once in a while, but not often or for very long.
4. Do not mind his/her being in the group, but not often or for very long.
5. Wish he/she were not in the group.

This procedures can be used as a classroom social distance scale to attempt to determine the general social tone of a particular class. Classroom social distance scores on each individual child can be obtained by arbitrarily weighting the items listed above. For example, if a child was checked two times for item number one (2 × 1 = 2); six times for item two (6 × 2 = 12); eight times for item three (8 × 3 = 24); three times for item four (3 × 4 = 12); and one time for item five (1 × 5 = 5) the total score would be 55. (The lower the score the greater acceptance by the group and the less social distance.)

These data can be used to determine, with some degree of objectivity, the extent to which certain school experiences have contributed to social relationships, that is, a teacher can compare scores before and after a group of children have been involved in a particular experience.

Over a period of years, I have used all of the above sociometric techniques with varying degrees of success. In some instances, the results have provided guidance in efforts to obtain a better understanding of social relationships and thus contribute to social health. It is recognized that all teachers are aware of those obvious factors concerned with social group structure. However, the many aspects of interpersonal relationships that are not so obvious can be difficult to discern. It is the purpose of sociometric techniques to assist in the emergence of these relationships.

HELPING CHILDREN LEARN ABOUT SOCIAL HEALTH

All teaching situations, whether during lessons devoted to health or not, should be such that the child has the opportunity to grow and to develop to a higher degree of social adjustment. The following concepts might serve as examples of some of the more significant aspects of social health.

Kindergarten

We share in school.
We wait and take turns.

Grade 1

Play can be more fun when we take turns and share.
We are a good sport when we play fair and follow the rules of the game.
It is important to be considerate of the wishes of others in our family.
School is a good place to make friends.
We are polite when we express our thanks for the kind things people do for us.

Grade 2

We help our family when we are considerate, kind, and cooperative.
When we do our share at home and school, we show we are growing up.
Adults can help us to make wise choices.

Grade 3

Each person can contribute something of interest to the group.
We help ourselves and others when we are good followers and good leaders.
Time can be saved by doing things together.
We need to assume our share of the responsibility for carrying out the plans we help to make.

Grade 4

Family life goes more smoothly and happily when all members share responsibilities.
Working in groups can make it easy to accomplish tasks that are hard to accomplish alone.
Having a friend and being a friend are important to happy group living.

Grade 5

People already living in a community can welcome or give help to newcomers.
Vacation time affords opportunities to develop new interests.

Grade 6

Growing up socially means growing in the ability to get along with others.

The ability to meet others graciously and to operate as a worthy group member help to make the individual pleasant company for others and add to his or her own happiness.

A good sport thinks of others as well as himself or herself.

Chapter 5

NUTRITION AND CHILD HEALTH

The 17th century gastronomist, Anthelme Brillat-Savarin, famous for his book, *The Physiology of Taste*, once said, "Tell me what you eat and I will tell you what you are." The more modern adage, "You are what you eat," could well have been derived from this old quotation. And, of course, it is true. Perhaps more so in modern times than was the case in the past. This old adage has been brought more clearly into focus recently because researchers now know that our bodies synthesize food substances known as *neurotransmitters*. Prominent nutritionists tend to be of the opinion that these neurotransmitters relay messages to the brain that, in turn, affect our moods, sex drives, appetite and even personality. This is to say that adding a certain food or omitting another could be just what a person might need.

At one time eating was fun and enjoyable; that is, until recent years when many of us have become victims of the "don't eat this, don't eat that" syndrome. The fact is that because certain aspects of nutrition and diet have become so controversial, many people in the general public have become more or less confused about the entire matter. It is the purpose of this chapter to attempt to clear up at least some of this confusion.

At the outset it should be stated very forcefully that any consideration of one's nutrition problems, eating habits, dietary concerns—of both children and adults—should be undertaken, if possible, with, or under the supervision of a physician and/or a qualified nutritionist.

NUTRITION

Nutrition can be described as the sum of the processes by which a person takes in and utilizes food substances; that is, the nourishment of the body by food. These processes consist of (1) ingestion, (2) digestion, (3) absorption, and (4) assimilation.

Ingestion derives from the Latin word *ingestus* meaning to take in, and in this context it means taking in food, or the act of eating. The process of *digestion* involves the breaking down or conversion of food into substances that can be *absorbed* through the lining of the intestinal tract and into the blood and used in the body. *Assimilation* is concerned with the incorporation or conversion of nutrients into *protoplasm* which is the essential material making up living cells.

Due to the fact that the body's needs change as it grows and develops, good nutrition for children is not the same as that for adults. In addition, to the nutrients needed to sustain their present status, children also need certain nutrients to help form new tissues. In her book on nutrition Jane Brody[1] estimates that a child of 5 weighing 44 pounds needs as much iron, calcium, and magnesium and even more vitamin D than a man of 25 who weighs 154 pounds. Although total quantities are smaller, pound for pound, 5 year olds need twice as much protein, thiamin, riboflavin, niacin, and vitamins A and C and three times as much B_6 and B_{12} as 25-year-old men. This means that the calories a child consumes need to be more densely packed with nutrients, but it does not mean that a young child should be eating as much food as an adult.

Growing children need plenty of certain minerals to build strong bones and teeth and protein for firm muscles as well as for energy and stamina. As a matter of fact, poorly nourished children will not be likely to grow properly. Thus, it is appalling that a recent report indicated that over 5 million children in the United States experience hunger every month. This is an atrocious record for a country that is supposed to be the so-called "land of plenty."

Essential Nutrients and Their Function in the Body

The body needs many nutrients or foods to keep it functioning properly. These nutrients fall into the broad groups of protein, carbohydrates, fats, vitamins, and minerals. (Although water is not a nutrient in the strictest sense of the word, it must be included, for nutrition cannot take place without it.)

Three major functions of nutrients are (1) building and repair of all body tissues, (2) regulation of all body functions, and (3) providing fuel for the body's energy needs. Although all of the nutrients can do their

---
[1] *Jane Brody's Nutrition Book*, New York, W. W. Norton & Company, 1981.

best work when they are in combination with other nutrients, each still has its vital role to play.

Protein

Protein is the protoplasmic matter from which all living animal cells and tissues are formed. It is the source of nitrogen, and it is from nitrogen that the building blocks of protein are formed. These basic substances are called *amino acids,* and they are to be found in plant and animal food sources.

The amino acids are acted upon and released during the digestive process, absorbed, and then rebuilt into new protein forms. For example, when a protein food such as meat is eaten, the digestive process promptly breaks it down into various amino acids. The body chemistry then goes to work to reassemble these amino acids into a new protein form. Some of the combinations are used to make cells for different tissues, such as muscle, blood, bone, and the soft tissues of the vital organs. Other amino acid combinations form the various hormones for the endocrine system, and still others are utilized to form enzymes. Enzymes are internal secretions necessary for the proper functioning of the blood, stomach, and other organs of the body. They are highly specialized and are responsible for such varied functions as aiding in the clotting of the blood and turning starches into sugar.

Some of the amino acids are used to make the brain chemicals or the previously-mentioned neurotransmitters. Three brain chemicals are *dopamine, norepinephrine,* and *serotonin.* An amino acid called *tyrosine* is of importance in the making of dopamine and norepinephrine, and *tryptophan.* According to Fathy Messiha, Professor of Pharmacology at the University of North Dakota, dopamine and norepinephrine are involved with increased muscle activity, more aggressive behavior and emotional states.

Protein is the basic raw material necessary for growth from the very beginning of life. It is necessary for the building of new tissue and the repairing of worn out tissue. It can also serve as a fuel for muscular work when needed, and we never outgrow our need for it. Since the metabolic process of the body is continuous, it is imperative that we have a continual supply of protein, so that the functions of the body can be successfully accomplished.

A body in the process of building itself—a growing child—needs a greater proportion of protein to weight than one that has reached its growth and uses protein only to repair worn out tissues. An average adult may require one gram of protein per kilogram of body weight daily, while a growing child may need two to three times this amount.

One source of protein for children is milk and nutritionists ordinarily recommend that a child drink a quart of milk daily. To be sure, for a growing child milk is an important source of protein as well as calcium and vitamin D. However, some children do not like milk, possibly because it may be forced upon them as the "perfect food." In addition, for one reason or another some children are allergic to milk and may lose their ability to digest it. Also there could perhaps be a risk of some children getting too much milk. This can possibly cause an iron deficiency and predispose a child to anemia due to the fact that milk is not a good source of iron.

Although most Americans obtain their protein from both plants and animal sources, certain religious groups, vegetarians, and people in countries where producing meat is not economically feasible have demonstrated that various plants provide many of the amino acids that are needed by man. Plants have the ability to synthesize all of the amino acids which they need for growth, but man is not self-sufficient. There are at least eight out of more than 25 amino acids necessary to man's health and growth which he is incapable of synthesizing satisfactorily from other foodstuffs. The amino acids which the body tissues cannot manufacture and must be obtained from outside sources are called "essential."

"Complete" protein foods are those which contain all of the essential amino acids. Animal meats are complete in this sense, as are also milk and milk products and eggs. Fish, too, are a good source of complete proteins. On the other hand, the fact is that large segments of the world population never eat meat and in some cases not even dairy products—but still grow into active adulthood. Thus it is clear that some vegetable foods likely provide all necessary proteins. Grain foods, nuts, peanuts, soy beans, peas and beans, and yeast are among the more important sources of nonanimal protein. Combinations of proteins seem to be especially valuable for meeting the body's needs.

Although proteins are essential for life, and are needed regularly, their importance should not lead to their being exaggerated in the diet. They are especially important during such times as when bodily tissues are being rebuilt following debilitating illnesses. Still, it is known that some people have gone without food of any kind for well over a week and have no ill effects. In other words, the comments concerning a continuous supply of protein or any other food should not lead one to think that they could not stand to miss an occasional meal, or several meals for that matter. After all, "three meals a day" is more of a conditioned response than a nutritional necessity. (This is particularly important as far as children are concerned because most of them need more than the three traditional meals daily.) It seems likely that the quality of one's food intake over a period of time—say several days—is more important than a meal-by-meal evaluation. However, efforts have been made by nutritionists to provide guidance as to what, roughly the body needs daily.

Carbohydrates

The carbohydrates which occur in our foods chiefly as sugar and starches are combinations of the chemical elements of carbon, hydrogen, and oxygen. These foods are broken down during the digestive process into simple sugars absorbed into the blood. It is from the blood that the tissues cells can withdraw sugar according to their energy needs.

Our main source of carbohydrates is foods composed of grains. These include breads and cereals (some of which are also rich in protein, minerals, and vitamins), spaghetti, macaroni, pastries, and the like. Potatoes are also a source of starch, but they contain other important food values as well.

Another important aspect of carbohydrates is that they provide fiber (once generally referred to as roughage), which adds bulk and helps to move the bowels. In recent years the lack of fiber in the diet has been of some concern because, on average, adults consume only about 40 percent of the fiber that is necessary. And some children may consume even less.

Generally speaking, usable carbohydrates have at least two fates in the body. The first is the formation of glucose. Glucose is the major energy source for the body and the only form of energy used by the brain, nerves, and lung tissue. One gram of carbohydrate yields four calories of energy. The second fate of carbohydrates is the formation of glycogen from glucose. Glycogen is a form of stored energy with the principal stores being in the liver. Smaller reserves are found in the muscles. Blood glucose comes from dietary complex carbohydrates and simple carbohydrates.

Fats

Fats are derived from the same chemical elements as carbohydrates but the combination of carbon, hydrogen, and oxygen is different. Fats contain more carbon but less oxygen than carbohydrates, and they are a more concentrated energy source than either carbohydrates or proteins. They also contribute to bodily functioning in other important ways and should not, therefore, be considered as substances to be completely eliminated from the diet.

Fat deposits in the body serve as insulation and shock absorption material and as reserve energy in storage. Individuals whose energy expenditure is likely to exceed that provided by their carbohydrate intake are especially in need of the "slower burning" fats in their diet. Individuals who wish or need to reduce their weight or who have certain circulatory disorders and risks usually are advised to restrict their fat intake more or less sharply. For several decades the consumption of fat has been about 40 percent of the diet. Because of the relationship to fat intake and heart disease in adults, it is generally recommended that on average the diet not exceed more than 30 percent fat. Incidentally, recent studies have found that children consume far too much fat, and this may be due to an excessive intake of the so-called "junk" foods.

Some people who consider themselves to be on a low fat diet sometimes wonder if they are getting too little fat. Although this is possible, it is not necessarily likely. For example, low fat foods such as chicken and fish contain some fat. Sometimes "strict dieters" may even avoid these foods because of their fat content. When one eliminates all animal protein and dairy foods they may have a diet that is too low in protein, iron, zinc, calcium, and other nutrients. A low fat diet is not necessarily a *no* fat diet. A diet containing 20 percent of calories from fat is considered as a low fat diet.

Fats are classified in two ways, saturated and unsaturated. Some sources of the former are meat fat, whole milk, butter, and cheese. With the exception of milk, some children will not have a great deal of fat in their diet. On the other hand, they might have an overabundance of carbohydrates due to the "sweet tooth" syndrome. Sources of unsaturated fats are most cooking oils and margarine, although recently the latter has become suspect. It is ordinarily recommended that unsaturated fats should be used in preference to saturated fats.

Minerals

The mineral elements of the body are often referred to as ash constituents, for they are the residue left from the oxidation process of the organic compounds which we eat in the form of food. In simpler terms, we may liken them to the ashes that remain after the burning of wood or coal. The mineral elements compose about four percent of the total body weight with calcium accounting for approximately 2 of the 4 percent.

Included among the minerals are calcium, phosphorous, potassium, sulfur, chlorine, sodium, magnesium, iron, iodine, manganese, copper, cobalt, nickel, and flourine. The majority of the minerals are needed in minute quantities that are plentiful in a good diet. However, calcium, iron, and iodine are needed in appreciable quantities and therefore may require special consideration in the diet. In the case of iron, it has already been mentioned that some children may be heavy milk drinkers and thus may suffer from the shortage of iron in milk. According to the previously-mentioned Jane Brody, adults with iron deficiency are not able to work as hard as they normally would, and children may have decreased attention span and decreased learning ability which disappear when proper levels of iron are restored.

As far as calcium is concerned some studies[2] suggest that children who boost their calcium intake develop significantly greater bone density. However true this may be, Ronald Kleiman, chairman of the American Academy of Pediatrics' Committee on Nutrition, cautions that there are potential risks from taking calcium supplements. For example, such side effects for children as stomach distress and constipation might occur. Parents who are considering providing a calcium supplement for their children should do so under the supervision of a pediatrician or qualified nutritionist.

The major function of minerals in the body is to serve as building and regulatory substances. As structural constituents, they operate in three general ways: (1) they give rigidity to the hard tissues of the bones and teeth, (2) they serve as components of soft tissues in muscle and nerve, and (3) they often serve as the crucial element necessary for the production of hormones such as iodine and thyroxin. As a regulator of body processes, minerals serve in many ways, examples of which are: (1) they (calcium) are essential for the coagulation of blood, (2) they protect against the accumulation of too much acid or alkali in the blood and

---

[2] Squires, Sally, More Calcium for Children, *Health, The Washington Post*, July 21, 1992.

body tissues, (3) they are involved in the maintenance of the normal rhythms of the heartbeat, (4) they aid in the exchange of water in the tissues, and (5) they are involved in the transmission of nerve impulses.

Minerals have an important and diverse use in human metabolism. Since many of them are required in carbohydrates, fat, and protein metabolism, they would be important in the energy reaction required during the stress response. However, it is important to take minerals in balanced proportions and not in excessive amounts since they can be toxic in high doses.

Vitamins

From an historical point of view, the realization that vitamins are basic nutrients stands as a milestone in the emergence of the field of nutrition as a scientifically-based discipline. Unlike such nutrients as proteins, fats, and carbohydrates, vitamins do not become a part of the structure of the body, but rather they serve as catalysts which make possible various chemical reactions within the body. The reactions have to do with converting food substances into the elements needed for utilization by the various cells of the body. For example, vitamin D needs to be present if calcium is to be metabolized and made available for use in the blood and bones.

The vitamins with which we are familiar today are commonly classified as fat soluble and water soluble. This designation means that the one group requires fatty substances and the other water if they are to be dissolved and used in the body. Although a large number of vitamins have been identified as being important to human nutrition, the exact function of many of them has not yet been clearly determined.

In countries such as the United States it should not be difficult for people to select a diet which is sufficiently varied to include all necessary vitamins. However, poor dietary practices can lead to vitamin inadequacy, and as a precaution many people supplement their diets with vitamin pills. Even though such a supplement may not be needed, when taken in small amounts the vitamins may do no harm. This is particularly true of the water soluble vitamins in that if one gets more than needed they will pass right through the body. (Recently, some scientists have been disputing this claim, especially if water soluble vitamins are taken in extra large doses). On the other hand, some of the fat soluble vitamins may be toxic and overdoses could render possible harm. Of course, extra vitamins may be prescribed by a physician for a variety of reasons.

Water

By far the greatest proportion of the body weight of human beings is water. This water, evaporating and flowing from the surface of the body, and breathed out as vapor on the breath, must be continuously replenished if one is to remain alive. The chemical changes which make life possible can take place only in solution, and it is water which provides the necessary solvent.

The body secures the water which it needs from fluids taken as drink, from foods which are eaten, and from the water formed by the combustion of foods in the body. The body loses water in the form of urine from the kidneys, fecal discharge from the intestinal tract, perspiration from the skin, and exhaled breath from the lungs.

Physical activity, environmental heat, and the normal bodily processes lead more or less rapidly to water loss. If this loss is not balanced by water intake, dehydration can occur. For short periods this loss is harmless and leads to thirst and restoration of normal water level and body weight with copious drinking. However, if the dehydrated state continues over an extended period of time, bodily functions become seriously jeopardized since water is involved in all of them.

A question that often arises is: How many glasses of water should we consume each day? Perhaps this should be considered in terms of liquids rather than water as such, because fruits and vegetables contain water. Recommendations of physicians are likely to vary on the amount of water intake one should have daily. Some will recommend that one start and end the day with an eight ounce glass of water with this same amount at each meal. Others suggest 6–8 glasses of water per day.

In fact, many such arbitrary recommendations have been made concerning the desirable intake per day. However, there are so many factors which affect the need for it—factors such as the fluid content of other liquids in food, how active a person is, and the environmental temperature—that one could be inclined to recommend thirst as a guide.

Calories

Many people labor under the misconception that a calorie is a nutrient just as fats, carbohydrates, or proteins. Actually, a calorie is a unit of measurement just like an ounce or an inch. The body requires energy to function and heat is the by-product of this energy. A calorie is the amount of heat necessary to raise the temperature of one kilogram (2.2

pounds) of water one degree centigrade. Since food is our source of fuel, scientists have been interested in computing the number of calories that different foods provide, as well as the number of calories that the body must utilize in the performance of various activities. The results of these studies have furnished information that tells us how many calories or heat units of food we eat must produce in order to provide us with enough energy to meet our needs. These energy needs may be classified into two categories, those that are voluntary and those that are involuntary. Voluntary activities are those over which we have control, but the involuntary energy demands are those which take place continuously whether we are awake or asleep. Among the latter are digestion, heart function, elimination, breathing, and such special demands automatically brought on by emotional excitation, stress, and environmental heat.

From infancy numerous people are actually trained to be especially fond of candies and dessert foods since these are used by parents as a reward for "cleaning up" one's plate, eating unwanted foods, and being "good" in other ways. In excess of bodily needs, such high energy foods have been termed "empty calories," because they provide little or nothing of value. Indeed, they well encourage fatness while at the same time satisfying the appetite when other food values are needed. It is not suggested that an effort be made to eliminate pastries and candies from the diet entirely, but an effort should be made to reduce their prominence. After all, fruits, vegetables, and juices can be equally satisfying foods (if prepared correctly) which are relatively low in calories and high in other nutrients, and they do not confront the body with the problem of disposing of pure, unneeded energy.

It is estimated that a one-year-old child consumes about 1,000 calories daily. By the age of three this rises to 1,300, and by age six, 1,700. (Consumption of excessive empty calories can elevate this number appreciably.) For the average adult male the amount of calories is 2,700, and the average adult female, 2,100.

Digestion

The digestive system of the body is more than 30 feet long from beginning to end, and the chemical processes that occur within the walls of this mucus-lined hollow tube are extremely complex in nature. From the moment that food is taken into the mouth until waste products are excreted, the body's chemical laboratory is at work. The principal parts of this system are the alimentary canal, consisting of the oral cavity, pharynx, esophagus, stomach, small intestine, and large intestine. Two additional organs are necessary to complete the digestive system. These are the liver and the pancreas, both of which connect to the small intestine. It is from these two organs that many of the essentially digestive juices are secreted.

As mentioned previously, the function of the digestive system is to change the composition of foods which we ingest. Reduced to simpler chemical substances, the foods can be readily absorbed through the lining of the intestines for distribution by the circulatory system to the millions of body cells. These end products of digestion are in the form of simple sugars, fatty acids, amino acids, minerals, and vitamins.

Digestion is also accomplished by mechanical action. First, the food is broken down by the grinding action of the teeth. (How many times as a child were you admonished to "chew your food and don't gulp it down?") This increases tremendously the food surface area upon which the various digestive juices can act. It is then swallowed and eventually is moved through the alimentary canal by a process called peristalsis. This is a series of muscular contractions, which mix the contents of the digestive tract and keep it on the move.

DIET

The term *diet* is an all inclusive one used to refer to foods and liquids regularly consumed. The question often raised is: "What constitutes a balanced diet?" This means essentially, that along with sufficient fluids, one should include foods from the *four basic food groups*. These are the dairy group, the meat group, the vegetable and fruit group, and the bread and cereal group.

A general recommendation is that children should receive daily three servings from the dairy group, two servings from the meat group, four or more servings from the fruit and vegetable group, and four or more servings from the bread and cereal group. Estimates of the size of a serving vary but Eva Hamilton and Eleanor Whitney[3] of Florida State University recommend that a child's serving be one tablespoon for each year of age. For example, a six-year-old child would receive six tablespoons for a serving. However, as mentioned previously the amounts can

---
3 Hamilton, Eva and Whitney, Eleanor, *Nutrition: Concepts and Controversies*, St Paul, West, 1979.

vary from one day to another. The problem may not be so much one of following an arbitrary diet, but one of learning to know on what foods and proportions of foods one functions best.

The diets of some families include too much of certain foods that can be potentially harmful. A case in point is the intake of *cholesterol.* Excessive amounts of this chemical component of animal oils and fats can be deposited in the blood vessels and may be a factor in the causation of hardening of the arteries leading to a heart attack.

There is no question about it, cholesterol has become one of the health buzzwords of the last decade. The importance of cholesterol as a risk factor prompted the First National Cholesterol Conference held November 9–11, 1988. This meeting was sponsored by the National Cholesterol Education Program Coordinating Committee which includes some 25 member organizations. This Conference was a somewhat unique forum in that the researchers, physicians, and policy and program experts shared knowledge and program successes in the rapidly changing field of cholesterol study.

The universal interest in this risk factor is certainly justified by such estimates as:

1. Over 50 percent of Americans have a cholesterol level that is too high.
2. Only about 8 percent of Americans know their cholesterol level.
3. As many as 250,000 lives could be saved each year if citizens were tested and took action to reduce their cholesterol levels.
4. For every 1 percent you lower your cholesterol, you reduce your risk of heart attack by 2 percent.
5. If your cholesterol level is 265 or over you have four times the risk of a heart attack as someone with 190 or less.
6. Nine out of ten people can substantially reduce their cholesterol by diet.

Physicians vary widely in their beliefs about the levels of cholesterol and not very long ago a very broad range of 150–300 was considered normal. However, recently thoughts on this matter have changed radically. For example the National Heart, Lung and Blood Institute has announced more stringent guidelines. That is, it is now believed that the total blood cholesterol should not exceed 200 (this means 200 milligrams of total cholesterol per deciliter of blood).

It is worthy of note that in his interesting book, *The Healing Heart,* the late Norman Cousins[4] suggested that the accumulation of these fatty substances is not something that begins in upper middle age. On the contrary, the process can begin in early childhood. A 1982–83 study of children in New York City and Los Angeles by Dr. Ernst L. Wynder of the American Heart Foundation showed average cholesterol levels of 180 for children in the 10–12 year age range. This is about 50 points above the normal for children of this age. Continuing on the same course would lead to cholesterol levels close to or above 300 by the age of 35. In this general regard it is interesting that the National Cholesterol Education Program suggests the following cholesterol intake for children as compared to adults.[5]

	Children	*Adults*
Acceptable	less than 170 mg/dl	less than 200 mg/dl
Borderline	170–199 mg/dl	200–239 mg/dl
High	Above 200 mg/dl	Above 240 mg/dl

CHILDREN'S EATING HABITS

Adult supervision, especially that of parents, is of utmost importance in children's eating habits. However, unfortunately in some cases some parents may be the child's worst enemy as far as eating habits are concerned. The nagging parent who tries to ply the child with foods that he or she may not like oftentimes can do a great deal of harm to the child's present and future eating habits.

At about the end of the first year of life children begin to have a rather remarkable change in their eating habits. For one thing, there is likely to be a large decrease in the intake of food. Many parents who do not understand the process of child development worry needlessly about this condition. What actually happens is that after the first year the growth rate of the child declines and as a consequence his or her need for calories per pound of body weight becomes less. This causes the appetite to decrease and this can vary from one meal to another, sometimes depending upon the kind and amount of activity in which the child engages. Thus, a parent who is aware of this will not expect the child of two or three years of age to eat the same way as when he or she was six months old. This knowledge for the parent is very important because he

---

4 Cousins, Norman, *The Healing Heart,* New York, W. W. Norton & Company, 1983.

5 Hart, Archibald D., *Stress and Your Child,* Wood Publishing Company, Dallas, 1992.

or she will not be so concerned with the *quantity* of the child's intake of food. This is to say that parents should be more concerned with *quality* of food than amount of intake.

Sometimes a child may develop a sudden like or dislike for certain foods. Reasons vary for this change in attitude. The child may want a particular cereal because of a prize in the box, and then may turn the food down because he or she is disenchanted and does not want the prize. Fortunately, more often than not, such likes and dislikes are not long-lasting, and adults should not worry too much about them.

It is a good practice to provide a rather large variety of foods early in the child's life. This helps to prevent a child from forming set opinions on food likes and dislikes. Adults should set an example by not allowing their own dislikes to influence children.

Adults often complain that a particular child is a "poor eater." When this occurs it is important to try to identify the cause of this problem. It may be that the child too frequently eats alone, and is deprived of the pleasant company of others. Or perhaps the portions are too large, particularly if it is felt that he or she must consume all of it. Mealtime should be a happy time. It is not a time for reprimanding and threatening if a child does not eat hardily. Such behavior on the part of adults can place the child under stress and create an eating problem that otherwise would probably not occur.

Some studies[6] of children in the 9-10 year old age range have found that these children were aware of foods that were *best* for health and those that were *worst* for health. Those foods identified as "best" were: vegetables, 36 percent; fruits, 28 percent; meat, 26 percent; bread, 8 percent; and somewhat surprisingly, milk only 2 percent. As for the "worst" foods for health: 65 percent said candy and other sweets; 17 percent said junk foods; 9 percent said salt; 5 percent said coffee; and 4 percent said fats. (This might well be a question of health knowledge and not necessarily health practice.)

In one interesting study[7] children in the 10-11 year age range were asked to name their favorite food. The results in order of preference were: pizza, hamburgers, spaghetti, ice cream, hot dogs, popcorn, and brownies. Of course, these results should not be interpreted to mean that

---

6 Humphrey, Joy N. and Humphrey, James H., *Child Development During the Elementary School Years*, Springfield, IL, Charles C Thomas Publisher, 1989.

7 Mini Page, *The Washington Post*, December 25, 1988.

these foods consist of a child's regular diet, but rather they are the foods they tend to like best. Nonetheless, a disturbing estimate is that Americans take as many as one-half of their meals out—and these out-of-home meals are likely to be taken at the "fast food" establishments. Singling out hot dogs in the above list, according to the National Hot Dog and Sausage Council—a trade association in Westchester, Illinois—Americans eat 50 million hot dogs a day, an average of 80 hot dogs per person per year. One of the problems with hot dogs is that there does not seem to be much good about them except taste. For example, the Center for Science in the Public Interest, A Washington, DC-based health advocacy group, claims that a typical 1½ ounce hot dog contains 13 grams of fat, 500 milligrams of sodium, and 145 calories. Moreover, about 80 percent of the calories are derived from fat and over ⅓ of this is saturated fat.

CHILDHOOD OBESITY

Obesity is due to excess storage of fat in the body. It is a serious hazard and can cause such serious disorders as diabetes and heart disease. For children, these health problems may be years away but it is some of the other things about obesity that can be devastating to the child. They may develop very negative feelings and loss of self-esteem and personal worth.

Although some cases of obesity may be caused by a glandular condition, by far the greatest majority are due to overeating. Stated simply, more calories are ingested than are necessary for energy and the excess food is stored in the body as fat.

According to Jane Brody[8] obesity tends to run in families. In families where both parents are of normal weight, only 7 percent of the children are overweight. But if one parent is fat, the chances of the children being fat as well leap to 40 percent. And if both parents are obese, 80 percent of the children are also likely to be obese. This suggests a strong hereditary tendency toward overweight, but it does not necessarily prove it. The family environment—especially the parents' eating and exercise habits—could also result in such statistics. In fact, although heredity was once considered of major importance in predicting a person's predilection for overweight, new evidence suggests that it plays a relatively minor role.

---
8 *Jane Brody's Nutrition Book,* New York, W. W. Norton & Company, 1981.

In addition, she also suggests that if a lifetime of obesity is not necessarily rooted in the genes, it must be influenced by events early in life. Indeed, early feeding patterns and attitudes toward food and eating can influence how much weight a child gains and how large his or her body's fat storage capacity gets to be. Fat is housed in special cells that can grow to be very large. Different people have different numbers of fat cells, which, once formed, remain in the body. As one loses weight or gains weight, the cells shrink or expand, but never diminish in number. The grossly obese adult who was obese as a child has on the average three times as many fat cells as his or her normal-weight counterpart, and the individual cells contain one and one-half times as much fat.

Childhood Obesity Research

In recent years a great deal of research has been conducted with obese children. Some representative examples of such studies are reported here.

Epstein and Associates[9] studied the effect of diet and controlled exercise on weight loss in obese children. The effects of adding exercise to diet for weight control in obese children were evaluated by randomizing obese girls to one of two groups: diet and diet plus exercise. During the first six weeks of the treatment, children exercised in a supervised three-times-a-week exercise program, in which they walked or ran three miles. Significant decreases from baseline weight and in percent overweight were observed for both groups during the year of treatment. Significant decreases in the percent overweight were observed at 0 to 2 months and then at 2 to 6 months for the children who were exercising, whereas percent overweight in children in the diet-alone group decreased only from 0 to 2 months. In addition, a significant improvement in fitness was observed only for children in the diet plus exercise group.

Epstein and other Associates[10] studied the long-term relationship between weight and aerobic-fitness change in children. The relationship between changes in relative weight and fitness was assessed five years after children began treatment for obesity. Multivariate regression analysis showed that two factors were independently related to fitness change:

---

9 Epstein, L. H., et al. Effect of Diet and Controlled Exercise on Weight Loss in Obese Children, *Journal of Pediatrics*, September 1985.

10 Epstein, L. H., et al. Long-term Relationship Between Weight and Aerobic-Fitness Change in Children, *Health Psychology*, 7 (1), 1988.

(1) maintenance of weight loss from the end of six months of treatment to the 5-year follow-up and (2) initial fitness level. Children who showed the largest long-term changes in relative weight and the lowest initial fitness showed the largest improvement in fitness. Short-term weight loss was not related to long-term fitness change. These results show that weight loss and fitness are related over 5 years.

Huttunen and Associates[11] explored physical activity and fitness in obese children. Daily physical activity and physical fitness were studied in 31 obese and 31 normal-weight children matched for age and sex. The ages of children ranged from 5.7 to 16.1 years. The history of their physical activity was examined using a questionnaire completed by the child and the parents. Physical fitness was measured using a two-stage exercise test on a bicycle ergometer. There were no significant differences in daily activities between the obese and the nonobese children, while the sports grades at school were lower and participation in the training teams of sports clubs was less frequent among obese than normal-weight subjects. The obese children were physically-less fit than the normal-weight subjects as judged from the pedalling time in the exercise test (P less than .05) and from the maximum oxygen consumption (VO_2 max) related to lean body mass (P less than .001). Twenty-seven children participated for one year in a weight-reduction program which comprised individual nutrition counselling, guidance of physical activities and supportive therapy. The reduction in weight was successful in 25 out of 27 children and VO_2 max increased on average from 44.2 to 47.1 ml/min/kg of lean body mass (P less than .025.). There was no change in the time used for physical activities during the weight reduction although the children's participation in the training teams of sports clubs increased. It was concluded that obese children are less fit than their nonobese counterparts.

Cooper and Associates[12] in an attempt to test the hypothesis that obese children are unfit (i.e., have abnormal responses to exercise testing consistent with reduced levels of habitual physical activity), used new analytic strategies in studies of 18 obese children performing cycle ergometry. The subjects' weight (mean +/− SD) was 168 +/− 24 percent that predicted by height, and the age range was 9 to 17 years. Size-

---

[11] Huttunen, N. P. et al, Physical Activity and Fitness in Obese Children, *International Journal of Obesity*, 10(6), 1986.

[12] Cooper, D. M., et al, Are Obese Children Truly Fit? Minimizing the Confounding Effect of Body Size on the Exercise Response, *Journal of Pediatrics*, February 1990.

independent measures of exercise (e.g., the ratio of oxygen uptake to work rate during progressive exercise and the temporal response of VO_2, carbon dioxide output (VCO_2, and minute ventilation (VE) at the onset of exercise) were used. The ability to perform external mechanical work was corrected for VO_2 at unloaded pedaling (change in maximum oxygen uptake (delta VO_2 max) and in anaerobic threshold (delta AT). On average, obese children's responses were in the normal range: delta VO_2 max, 104 +/− 41 percent (+/− SD) predicted (by age); delta AT, 85 +/− 51 percent; ratio of change VE to change in work rate, 100 +/− 24 percent, but six of the obese children had values of delta VO_2 max or delta AT that were more than 2 SD below normal. In addition, obese children did not have increased delta VO_2 max or delta AT with age as observed in nonobese children. Although the response time of VO_2 was normal (99 +/− 32 percent of predicted), those for both VCO_2 and VE were prolonged. It was concluded that the finding of obesity in a child is not a reliable indicator of poor fitness but that testing cardiorespiratory responses to exercise can be used to identify subjects with serious impairment and to individualize therapy.

Recently, studies are showing that children as young as five years of age who are fat and unfit may be at risk for high blood pressure. Specific reference is made to the research of Dr. Bernard Gutin[13] with five- and six-year-old inner-city children in New York. Fitness was judged by measuring how hard the children had to work on a treadmill, and fatness was determined by using calipers to measure skin folds of weight proportionate to height. A statistical analysis of the measurements indicated that as fitness decreased and fatness increased, blood pressure rose.

Finally, writing in the foreword of one of my recent books,[14] Dr. Paul J. Rosch commented that, "Protracted television watching has also been linked to obesity and elevated cholesterol, possibly because of associated fast food snacking and/or increased secretion of stress related hormones. Over the past two decades, morbid childhood obesity has increased over 50%."

---

[13] Gutin, Bernard, et al., Blood Pressure and Fatness in 5- and 6-year-old Children, *The Journal of the American Medical Association*, September 5, 1990.

[14] Humphrey, James H., *Stress Management For Elementary Schools*, Springfield, Il, Charles C Thomas Publisher, 1993.

HELPING CHILDREN LEARN ABOUT FOODS AND NUTRITION

Many elementary schools make an attempt to teach children about foods and nutrition. This may be done through a specific curriculum in health education or in units in foods and nutrition as a part of the science or social studies curriculum. Whatever way it is done, an attempt is made to provide a sequence of food and nutrition concepts that children can internalize at the respective grade levels.

In kindergarten the emphasis is upon the practice of starting the day with a good breakfast and eating a good lunch and dinner. Stress in the first grade is on good eating practices and the importance of foods. The second-grade content carries the emphasis of the kindergarten and first grade, with the addition of selection and variety of foods. General foods such as meats, fruits and vegetables, milk and milk products, and bread and cereals are introduced. Third-grade content deepens the previous concepts, adds care and handling of foods, and introduces the idea of what foods do for the body. At the upper elementary level the subject matter should be much more structured. The four food groups are introduced in the fourth grade; elements of food, in the fifth grade; and the body's dependence upon foods, in the sixth grade. Following are some suggested concepts that might be developed.

Kindergarten

We choose a good breakfast.
We drink milk every day.
We drink water every day.
We eat a good lunch.
We eat a good dinner.
We eat a snack.

Grade 1

The food we eat helps us to grow big and strong and to keep well.
To be healthy we need to eat breakfast, lunch, and dinner every day.
Milk helps us grow.
We need to drink enough water every day.
Fruit makes a good after school snack.
Breakfast can help to keep us happy and wide awake.

Grade 2

Some foods that help us grow strong and healthy are meats, fruits and vegetables, milk and milk products, and bread and cereal.
Food from breakfast helps give us energy to work and play in the morning.
As healthy children we will want to try to eat well-balanced meals each day.
We should select and eat a variety of foods every day.
Milk helps us grow strong and healthy.
Good food helps our teeth grow.
It is good for our bodies to have water every day.
We should eat slowly and chew our food well.

Grade 3

Proper food gives us energy, and builds strong muscles, teeth, and bones.
Good food helps the body keep well and fight disease.
It is a good idea to eat regular meals and to select a variety of foods to be healthy.
Sweets between meals can take away our appetite.
Milk helps our teeth to grow strong.
Unless proper care is taken food will spoil and become unfit to eat.
Special care is needed in the handling of food at the store and in the home to keep it clean, fresh, and free from germs.
Pasteurization kills germs in milk and makes it safer to drink.
People who handle food should be clean, especially their hands.
Clean food is best for good health.
We need to drink safe pure water.

Grade 4

There are four groups of foods important to good health.
It is good for the body to have a daily supply of foods from each of the four food groups for good nutrition.
Fruits and vegetables help our bodies to grow and maintain good health.
Milk and milk products give us energy, make good teeth and bones, and help our bodies to grow.
Meat, fish and eggs can give our bodies the materials needed for muscles and blood.

Bread, cereal, butter, and margarine give our bodies heat and energy.
Our bodies need and use the water we drink.
Food supplies energy and a lack of proper food can make us tired.

Grade 5

The cells in our body get their nourishment from the materials in foods called food elements.
Food can keep us well, help us grow, give heat and energy to the body, and protect us from disease.
The food elements are carbohydrates, fats, protein, minerals, and vitamins.
Almost all foods are a mixture of several different elements.
Carbohydrates (starch and sugar) and fats (vegetable and animal) furnish heat and energy.
Proteins (primarily from meat, milk, eggs, and fish) are important for the building, repair, and maintenance of body cells.
Minerals (from plant-eating animals) help regulate certain body functions and furnish the calcium necessary for bone formation.
Vitamins help our bodies use all the other elements of foods.
Vitamins help to regulate body function and to protect our health.
Vitamins A and B help strengthen the eyes and keep the skin healthy and the hair glossy.
Vitamin B helps steady nerves and aids in digestion.
Vitamin D (sunshine vitamin) helps calcium and phosphorus to build bones and teeth.
Our body uses water for carrying on body functions.
When we eat properly we show we are learning to care for our bodies.

Grade 6

Body cells are dependent upon the wise choice of foods.
Since no single food contains all essentials, the cells of the body require a supply of the four basic food elements.
The amount of food required daily depends upon how active a person is and the quantity of energy used by the body.
Water helps carry food to the cells and to carry waste away from them.
Bacteria, which decays food, is destroyed or its growth is prevented by methods used to preserve foods (canning, pasteurization, refrigeration, and drying).

Careful methods of production, handling, purchasing, and storage should be used to keep foods free from harmful bacteria.

Families can protect their food supply by refrigeration, clean utensils, and sanitary surroundings.

Good nutrition depends upon adequate digestion as well as an ample supply of basic food elements.

As food is used in the body, it provides necessary heat and energy.

The need for energy is constant because the body never stops working.

We can help one another to make mealtime more enjoyable by being punctual and by using good table manners.

Eating with others can be an enjoyable social experience.

These concepts are suggestive and others may be added, depending upon the needs in a given local situation.

Chapter 6

BODY RESTORATION AND CHILD HEALTH

In the present context *body restoration* means the relief of and/or the recovery from fatigue through the process of rest, sleep and relaxation.

To be effective and to enjoy life to the utmost, periodic recuperation is an essential ingredient in the daily living patterns of all of us—adults as well as children. Rest, sleep, and relaxation provide us with the means of revitalizing ourselves to meet the challenges of our responsibilities.

FATIGUE

In order to keep fatigue at a minimum and in its proper proportion in the cycle of everyday activities, nature has provided us with ways to help combat and reduce it. First, however, we should consider what fatigue is so that it may then be easier for us to cope with it. There are two types of fatigue, *acute* and *chronic*.

Acute Fatigue

Acute fatigue is a natural outcome of sustained or severe exertion. It is due to such physical factors as the accumulation of by-products of muscular exertion in the blood and to excessive "oxygen debt"—the inability of the body to take in as much oxygen as is being consumed by muscular work. Psychological considerations may also be important in acute fatigue. That is, an individual who becomes bored with what he or she is doing and who becomes preoccupied with the discomfort involved will become "fatigued" much sooner than if highly motivated to do the same thing, is not bored, and does not think about the discomfort.

Activity that brings on distressing acute fatigue in one individual may amount to mild, even pleasant, exertion in another. The difference in fatigue level is due essentially to the physical fitness; that is, training of the individual for particular activities under consideration. Thus, a good walker or dancer may soon become fatigued when running or swimming hard. The key, then to controlling acute fatigue is sufficient training in the activities to be engaged in to prevent premature and undue fatigue. Knowing one's limits at any given time is also important as a guide to avoiding excessively fatiguing exertion and to determining what preparatory training is necessary. Adults must be on the lookout for any fatigue symptoms in children.

Chronic Fatigue

Chronic fatigue has reference to fatigue which lasts over extended periods—in contrast to acute fatigue, which tends to be followed by a recovery phase and restoration to "normal" within a more or less brief period of time. Chronic fatigue may be due to any and a variety of medical conditions ranging from a disease to malnutrition (such conditions are the concern of the physician who, incidentally, should evaluate all cases of chronic fatigue to assure that a disease condition is not responsible). It may also be due to psychological factors such as extreme boredom and/or worry about having to do, over an extended period, what one does not wish to do.

REST

In general, most people think of rest as just "taking it easy." A chief purpose of rest is to reduce tension so that the body may be better able to recover from fatigue. There is no overt activity involved, but neither is there loss of consciousness as in sleep. In rest, there is not loss of awareness of the external environment as in sleep. Since the need for rest is usually in direct proportion to the type of activity in which we engage, it follows naturally that the more strenuous the activity, the more frequent the rest periods should be. A busy day at school may not be as noticeable as a game of tennis, nevertheless, it is the wise person who will let the body dictate when a rest period is required. Five or ten minutes of sitting in a chair with eyes closed may make the difference in the course of an active day. The real effectiveness of rest periods for children depend largely on the individual child and his or her ability to let down and rest.

SLEEP

Sleep is a phenomenon that has never been clearly and completely defined or understood but it has aptly been named the "great restorer." And an old Welsh proverb states that "Disease and sleep keep far apart." It is no wonder that authorities on the subject agree that sleep is essential to the vital functioning of the body and that natural sleep is the most satisfying form of recuperation from fatigue. It is during the hours of sleep that the body is given an opportunity to revitalize itself. All vital functions are slowed down so that the building of new cells and the repair of tissues can take place without undue interruption. This does not mean that the body builds and regenerates tissue only during sleep, but it does mean that it is the time that nature has set aside to accomplish the task more easily. The body's metabolic rate is lowered and energy is restored.

Throughout the ages many theories about sleep have been advanced. The ancient Greeks believed that sleep was the result of the blood supply to the brain being reduced. A later idea about sleep was based on the research conducted by the Russian scientist Ivan Pavlov. That is, that sleep was an aspect of *conditioned reflex*. According to this theory the brain is "conditioned" and respond to any stimulus to become more active. And, the brain can develop the habit of reacting to certain stimuli with the slowing down of the activity. This means that when one is in an environment associated with sleep (bedroom) the brain gets a signal to start to slow down and finally one goes to sleep.

This theory was followed by one that suggested that while awake the body stored up waste products that tended to dull the higher centers of the brain, thus causing one to sleep.

In more modern times scientists are of the opinion that sleep occurs in cycles and each of these cycles, which are one and one-half to two hours in length, a sleeper uses about 75 percent of this time in what is called S sleep. This is concerned with what are referred to as Delta brain waves in which one is in deep sleep. The second stage is known as D sleep. At this time one may be in deep sleep but at the same time some parts of the nervous system are active and there are *rapid eye movements* (REM). The theory is that S sleep restores the body physically and D sleep restores it psychically. Whatever the theory of sleep, it has been suggested recently that on average we do not get enough of it. For example, Richard Allen, Codirector of the Johns Hopkins University Sleep Disorder Center, has been quoted as saying: "There's a fairly pervasive lack of adequate sleep in our society, which leads to problems with alertness and life satisfaction." And further that, "The quantity of wakefulness may be increased but the quality is decreased."[1]

Despite the acknowledged need for sleep, a question of paramount importance concerns the amount of sleep necessary for the body to accomplish its recuperative task. There is no clear-cut answer to this query. Sleep is an individual matter, based on degree rather than kind. The usual recommendation for adults is eight hours of sleep out of every 24, but the basis for this could be one of fallacy rather than fact. There are many persons who can function effectively on much less sleep, while others require more. (This is, of course, higher for children at the different age levels.) No matter how many hours of sleep one gets during the course of a 24-hour period, the best test of adequacy is how one feels. If one is normally alert, feels healthy, and in good humor he or she is probably getting a sufficient amount of sleep. The rest that sleep usually brings to the body depends to a large extent upon a person's freedom from excessive emotional tension and ability to relax. Unrelaxed sleep has little restorative value, but learning to relax is a skill that is not acquired in one night.

Is loss of sleep dangerous? This is a question that is pondered quite frequently. Again, the answer is not simple. To the normally healthy person with normal sleep habits, an occasional missing of the accustomed hours of sleep is not serious. On the other hand, repeated loss of sleep over a period of time can be dangerous. It is the loss of sleep night after night, rather than at one time, that apparently does the damage and results in the condition previously described as chronic fatigue. The general effects of loss of sleep are likely to result in poor general health, nervousness, irritability, inability to concentrate, lower perseverance of effort, and serious fatigue. Alert teachers can quickly discern those children who are getting an insufficient amount of sleep at home.

Studies have shown that a person can go for much longer periods of time without food than without sleep. In some instances successive loss of sleep for long periods have proven fatal. Under normal conditions, however, a night of lost sleep followed by a period of prolonged sleep will restore the individual to his or her normal self.

There are many conditions that tend to rob the body of restful slumber.

---

[1] Streitfeld, David. And so to Bed . . . but not Necessarily to Sleep, *The Washington Post*, April 26, 1988.

Most certainly, mental anguish and worry play a very large part in holding sleep at bay. Some factors that influence the quality of sleep are hunger, cold, boredom, and excessive fatigue. In many instances these factors can be controlled. Incidentally, Robert Coursey, a psychologist at the University of Maryland and a researcher of sleep, has indicated that people who are "insomniacs" may only think they are, and one of the things that insomniacs worry about incessively is their sleepless condition. His definition of a chonic insomniac is one who takes longer to fall asleep, has more trouble staying asleep, wakes up earlier than a normal sleeper, and feels tired as a result. In any case, insomnia and chronic fatigue might well be brought to the attention of a physician so that the necessary steps can be taken to bring about restoration of normal sleep patterns. Certainly, drugs to induce sleep should be utilized only if prescribed by a physician.

Some recommendations about sleep might include (1) relaxing physically and mentally before retiring, (2) reducing tension levels during the day, (3) managing one's time, activities, and thoughts to prepare for a good night's sleep, and (4) the process should be the same each night, and should begin at the same hour, leading to repose at the same hour. That is, if one's bedtime is normally eleven o'clock, preparation should perhaps begin at least by ten and probably not later than ten-thirty.

CHILDREN'S SLEEP HABITS

During the first year of a child's life it is a common practice to have two nap periods, one in the morning and one in the afternoon. The year-old child ordinarily, but gradually, gives up the morning nap and this tends to increase the afternoon nap time as well as the night sleep. With age the child will decrease the afternoon nap time and as a consequence will sleep longer at night. Although there is some difference of opinion on when a child should give up both the morning and afternoon nap, it is generally considered that preschoolers should have at least one nap a day, preferably in the afternoon.

As in the case of adults, school-age children differ in the number of hours of sleep required. The general recommendation is that on average out of every 24 hours they should get ten hours of sleep. A very important factor is that bedtime be a happy time. Parents should not make an issue of it so that conflict results. Perhaps a good rule for a younger child is that he or she be "taken" to bed rather than "sent." The ceremony of reading or telling the child a pleasant story at bedtime is important and can help lessen the impact of sudden separation. It is important to remember that some of the sleep disorders of children such as nightmares and bed wetting can be traced directly to stressful conditions under which separation at bedtime occurs.

RELAXATION

Learning to relax as a child could be as important to life in the future as many other things learned at home and in school. Indeed, most children need some sort of relaxation to relieve the tensions encountered during the school day.

THE MEANING OF RELAXATION AND RELATED TERMS

One derivation of the term *relax* is from the Latin word *relaxare*, meaning "loosen." It is interesting that a rather common parting comment among some people is the admonishment to "stay loose"—no doubt good advice.

The reality of muscle fibers is that they have a response repertoire of one. All they can do is contract, and this is the response they make to the electrochemical stimulation of impulses carried via the motor nerves. *Relaxation* is the removal of this stimulation.[2]

The terms *relaxation, refreshment,* and *recreation* are often confused in their meaning. Although all of these factors are important to the well-being of the human organism, they should not be used interchangeably to mean the same thing. *Refreshment* is the result of an improved blood supply to the brain for "refreshment" from central fatigue and to the muscles for the disposition of their waste products. This explains in part why muscular activity is good for overcoming the fatigue of sitting quietly (seventh inning stretch) and for hastening recovery after strenuous exercise (an athlete continuing running for a short distance slowly after a race).

Recreation may be described as the experience from which a person emerges with the feeling of being "re-created." No single activity is sure to bring this experience to all members of the group, nor is there assurance that an activity will provide recreation again for a given

---
[2] Brown, Barbara B., *Stress and the Art of Biofeedback*, New York, Bantam Books, Inc., 1978.

person because it did so the last time. These are more the marks of a psychological than a physiological experience. An important essential requirement for a recreational activity is that it completely engross the individual; that is, it must engage his or her entire individual attention. It is really escape from the disintegrating effects of distraction to the healing effect of totally integrated activity. Experiences that produce this effect may range from a hard game of tennis to the reading of a comic strip.[3]

Some individuals consider recreation and relaxation to be one and the same thing, which is not the case. Recreation can be considered a type of mental diversion that can be helpful in relieving tension. Although mental and muscular tensions are interrelated, it is in the muscle that the tension state is manifested.

LEARNING HOW TO RELAX

For many years, recommendations have been made with regard to procedures that might be applied in order to relax the muscles. In consideration of any technique designed to accomplish relaxation, one very important factor that needs to be taken into account is that learning to relax the muscles is a skill. That is, it is a skill based on the kinesthetic awareness of the feelings of *tonus* (the normal degree of contraction present in most muscles, which keeps them always ready to function when needed). Unfortunately, it is a skill that very few of us practice—probably because we have little awareness of how to go about it.

One of the first steps in learning to relax the muscles is to experience tension. That is, one should be sensitive to tensions that exist in his or her body. This can be accomplished by voluntarily contracting a given muscle group, first very strongly and then less and less. Emphasis should be placed on detecting the signal of tension as the first step in "letting go" (relaxing).

You might wish to try the traditional experiment used to demonstrate this phenomenon. Raise one arm so that the palm of the hand is facing outward away from your face. Now, bend the wrist backward and try to point the fingers back toward your face and down toward the forearm. You should feel some *strain* at the wrist joint. You should also feel

---

[3] Steinhaus, Arthur, *Toward an Understanding of Health and Physical Education,* Dubuque, Iowa, Wm. C. Brown Publishers, 1963.

something else in the muscle and this is tension, which is due to the muscle contracting the hand backward. Now, flop the hand forward with the fingers pointing downward and you will have accomplished a tension-relaxation cycle.

As in the case of any muscular skill, learning how to relax takes time and one should not expect to achieve complete satisfaction immediately. After one has identified a relaxation technique that he or she is comfortable with, increased practice should eventually achieve satisfactory results.

PROGRESSIVE RELAXATION

So that the reader will have an understanding of how to progressively relax the various muscle groups, this technique is discussed here. This technique was developed by Edmund Jacobson many years ago and is still the one most often referred to in the literature and probably the one that has had the most widespread application. In this technique, the person concentrates on progressively relaxing one muscle group after another. The technique is based on the procedure of comparing the difference between tension and relaxation. That is, as previously mentioned, one senses the feeling of tension in order to get the feeling of relaxation. In suggesting the use of the technique with children, Jacobson[4] indicates that for them, instructions in how to recognize the experience of contraction in various muscles could be to a large extent omitted.

In progressive relaxation, one of the first steps is to be able to identify the various muscle groups and how to tense them so that tension and relaxation can be experienced. However, before making suggestions on how to tense and relax the various muscle groups, there are certain preliminary measures that need to be taken into account.

1. You must understand that this procedure takes time and, like anything else, the more you practice the more proficient you should become with the skills.
2. The particular time of day is important and this is pretty much an individual matter. Some recommendations suggest that progressive relaxation be practiced daily—sometimes during the day and again in the evening before retiring. For many people this would be difficult unless one time period was set aside before going to

---
4 Jacobson, Edmund, *You Must Relax*, 4th ed., New York, McGraw-Hill, 1962.

the job in the morning. This might be a good possibility and might help a person to start the day relaxed.
3. It is important to find a suitable place to practice the tensing-relaxing activities. Again, this is an individual matter, with some preferring a couch and others a comfortable chair.
4. Consideration should be given to the amount of time a given muscle is tensed. You should be sure that you are able to feel the difference between tension and relaxation. This means that tension should be maintained from about four to not more than eight seconds. (This could be contraindicated for persons with hypertension.)
5. Breathing is an important concomitant in tensing and relaxing muscles. To begin with, it is suggested that three or more deep breaths be taken and held for about five seconds. This will tend to make for better rhythm in breathing. Controlled breathing makes it easier to relax and it is most effective when it is done deeply and slowly. It is ordinarily recommended that one should inhale deeply when the muscles are tensed and exhale slowly when "letting go."

How to Tense and Relax Various Muscles

Muscle groups may be identified in different ways. The classification given here consists of four different groups: (1) muscles of the head, face, tongue, and neck, (2) muscles of the trunk, (3) muscles of the upper extremities, and (4) muscles of the lower extremities.

Muscles of the Head, Face, Tongue and Neck

There are two chief muscles of the head, the one covering the back of the head and the one covering the front of the skull. There are about 30 muscles of the face, including muscles of the orbit and eyelids, mastication, lips, tongue, and neck.

Muscles in this group may be tensed and relaxed as follows (relaxation is accomplished by "letting go" after tensing):

1. Raise the eyebrows by opening the eyes as wide as possible. You might wish to look into a mirror to see if you have formed wrinkles on the forehead.
2. Tense the muscles on either side of the nose like you were going to sneeze.
3. Dilate or flare out the nostrils.

4. Force an extended smile from "ear to ear" at the same time clenching your teeth.
5. Pull one corner of your mouth up and then the other up as in a "villainous sneer."
6. Draw your chin up as close to your chest as possible.
7. Do the opposite of the above, trying to draw your head back as close to your back as possible.

Muscles of the Trunk

Included in this group are the muscles of the back, chest, abdomen, and pelvis. Here are some ways you can tense some of these muscles.

1. Bring your chest forward and at the same time put your shoulders back with emphasis on bringing your shoulder blades as close together as possible.
2. Try to round your shoulders and bring your shoulder blades far apart. This is pretty much the opposite of the above.
3. Give your shoulders a shrug, trying to bring them up to your ears at the same time as you try to bring your neck downward.
4. Breathe deeply and hold it momentarily and then blow out the air from your lungs rapidly.
5. Draw in your stomach so that your chest is out beyond your stomach. Exert your stomach muscles by forcing out to make it look like you are fatter than you are.

Muscles of the Upper Extremities

This group includes muscles of the hands, forearms, upper arms, and shoulders. A number of muscles situated in the trunk may be grouped with the muscles of the upper extremities, their function being to attach the upper limbs to the trunk and move the shoulders and arms. In view of this, there is some overlapping in muscles groups *two* and *three*. Following are some ways to tense some of these muscles.

1. Clench the fist and then open the hand, extending the fingers as far as possible.
2. Raise one arm shoulder high and parallel to the floor. Bend at the elbow and bring the hand in toward the shoulder. Try to touch your shoulders while attempting to move the shoulder away from the hand. Flex your opposite biceps in the same manner.

3. Stretch one arm out to the side of the body and try to point the fingers back toward the body. Do the same with the other arm.
4. Hold the arm out the same way as above, but this time have the palm facing up and point the fingers inward toward the body. Do the same with the other arm.
5. Stretch one arm out to the side, clench the fist and roll the wrist around slowly. Do the same with the other arm.

Muscles of the Lower Extremities

This group includes muscles of the hips, thighs, legs, feet, and buttocks. Following are some ways to tense some of these muscles.

1. Hold one leg out straight and point the toes as far forward as you can. Do the same with the other leg.
2. Do the same as above but point the toes as far backward as you can.
3. Turn each foot outward as far as you can and release. Do just the opposite by turning the foot inward as far as you can.
4. Try to draw the thigh muscles up so that you can see the form of the muscles.
5. Make your buttocks tense by pushing down if you are sitting in a chair. If you are lying down try to draw the muscles of the buttocks in close by attempting to force the cheeks together.

The above suggestions include several possibilities for tensing various muscles of the body. As you practice some of these, you will also discover other ways to tense and then let go. A word of caution might be that, in the early stages, you should be alert to the possibility of cramping certain muscles. This can happen particularly with those muscles that are not frequently used. This means that at the beginning you should proceed carefully. It might be a good idea to keep a record or diary of your sessions so that you can refer back to these experiences if this might be necessary. This will also help you to get into each new session by reviewing your experiences in previous sessions.

USING RELAXATION WITH CHILDREN

Clinical experience and empirical research with adults suggests that relaxation training might be an effective intervention for reducing and possibly preventing stress-related problems in children. The need for an evaluation of relaxation training with children is clear, particularly with increased prescription of relaxation as an intervention for a variety of child problems ranging from hyperactivity to asthma.

The research suggests that the results clearly support the labeling of relaxation training as the "aspirin" of behavior therapy for children as well as for adults. Relaxation training has been applied to numerous topographically and functionally different problems and in all cases has enhanced performance, has reduced behavioral distress, or has no effect at all. It has never been found to be harmful.[5]

Progressive Relaxation for Children

The relaxation techniques used with children follow the same theory of relaxation used with adults; that is, the purpose is to experience tension in a muscle or group of muscles and then "let go."

Some attempts have been made to modify Jacobson's progressive relaxation technique for children. Notable in this regard is the prominent California Psychologist, Stewart Bedford[6] who has made the following recommendations in his excellent book for children.

1. Find a comfortable place to relax. You can do it lying down or on a bed or the floor. You can do it in a recliner or sitting in a chair. If you practiced relaxing in different positions, it will be easier for you to transfer this training into your life in general. After you have learned to relax, you will probably want to relax in more than one way and in more than one place. If you relax sitting down, it will be easier to relax while sitting at your desk. If you relax while lying down, it will be easier to go to sleep when you want to.
2. Don't wear shoes or tight clothes. It's best to be warm but not too hot.
3. When you get yourself into a comfortable position, take a deep breath. Fill your lungs with air while you count slowly to ten. Then let the air out—all out. Concentrate on how your lungs feel when they are full of air and how they feel when they are empty.
4. Now think about your hands. Tense the muscles in your hands.

---
5 Armstrong, F. D., Collins, F. L. and Walker, C Eugene, Relaxation Training with Children: A Review of the Literature, in *Human Stress: Current Selected Research*, Vol. 2 New York, AMS Press, Inc, 1988, Ed. James H. Humphrey.

6 Bedford, Stewart, *Stress and Tiger Juice*, Chico, CA, Scott Publications, 1980.

Make fists. Think about how your hands feel when they are tense. Hold the tension while you count slowly to ten. Now relax the muscles in your hands and think about how they feel when they are relaxed. Concentrate on how your hands feel.
5. Now tense the muscles of your shoulders and arms. Think about how tense these muscles feel when they are tense. Hold this tension while you count slowly to ten. Now relax and think about how the muscles feel when they are relaxed. Get acquainted with your tense feelings. Get acquainted with your relaxed feelings. Learn how your body feels.
6. Now tense the muscles of your forehead. Raise your eyebrows as high as you can and think about how your face feels (think about how your face *feels*, not how it looks). Count slowly to ten and then relax. Now think about how these muscles feel when they are relaxed. Remember, think about the muscles when they are tense and when they are relaxed.
7. Now tense the muscles of your jaws. Clamp your teeth together and concentrate on how the muscles feel. Count slow to ten and then relax. Now think about the muscles of your jaws when they are relaxed.
8. Take another deep breath. Hold the air in while you count slowly to ten. Think about your chest. Let the air out slowly and relax. Think about your chest when it is relaxed.
9. Arch your back a little and tense your back muscles. Hold the tension and think about it while you count slowly to ten. Now relax and think about the back muscles when they are relaxed.
10. Tighten the muscles of your stomach. Pretend that someone is going to sock you with a ball and you are going to brace yourself so it doesn't hurt. Concentrate on the tight muscles. Count slowly to ten. Relax. Think about the muscles in your stomach when they are relaxed.
11. Tense the muscles in both legs and feet. Hold the tension while you count slowly to ten. Think about the muscles when they are relaxed.
12. Now, try to relax all the muscles in your body. Get as comfortable as you can. Concentrate on your breathing. Think about the air coming into your body and going out of your body. Air coming in. Air going out. Concentrate on your breathing. Breathe deeply. Breathe slowly. Practice letting your stomach muscles pull the air

in and push the air out. Concentrate on this and do this kind of breathing for about five minutes. If you start thinking about other ideas, pull your thoughts back to your breathing. Air coming in. Air going out. Air coming in. Air going out.

12. If you go to sleep while doing this part of the exercise, don't worry. If you stay awake, you will get more good out of the relaxation, but a little sleep doesn't hurt us now and then. If you do these activities twice a day, you will gradually learn how to get into deep muscle relaxation. When you have learned how to control relaxation in your muscles, you have learned one of the methods of managing your stress energies. You have learned a little more about the control of your emergency reaction. Remember, it is hard to be tense and relaxed at the same time.

Others have used versions of progressive relaxation with children. For example, two of my collaborators on a writing project, psychologists John Carter and Harold Russell,[7] have developed a series of tapes for child relaxation. One of these is patterned after the idea of progressive relaxation and involves tensing and relaxing various muscle groups. This is to help make the children aware of their own muscular tension and to learn how it feels to release their tensions. In the following sequence children are asked to tense for five seconds and then to relax and feel the tension leaving for ten seconds.

1. Squeeze your eyes shut—tightly—hold it, relax.
2. Push your lips together, very tightly—hold it, relax.
3. Press your tongue to the roof of your mouth—hold it, relax.
4. Shrug your shoulders up toward your ears—hold it—relax—feel the tension leaving.
5. With both hands make a fist as tight as you can—feel the tension building—relax. Feel the tension leaving.
6. Make a fist with your right hand. Notice the difference between your tense right hand and your relaxed left. Relax your right hand.
7. Make a fist with your left hand. Feel the left hand getting tense while your right hand is relaxing—relax your left hand.
8. Pull your stomach way in toward your backbone—hold it—relax—feel the tension leaving.

---
[7] Carter, John L., and Russell, Harold, Use of Biofeedback Relaxation Procedures with Learning Disabled Children, in *Stress in Childhood*, New York, AMS Press, Inc., 1984, ed. James H. Humphrey.

9. Push your knees together—hard—hold it. Relax.
10. Pull your toes toward your knees, way up. Hold it, relax. Feel the tension leaving your legs.
11. Point your toes. Hold it—relax.
12. Now tighten every muscle in your body—hold it—relax your entire body. Let your entire body get very limp—relaxed and comfortable.

When this is completed, breathing instructions are presented. The children are asked to breathe in through their nose and out through their mouth. They are asked to do this naturally and rhythmically. Each time they breathe out, they are reminded to let themselves get just a little more limp, a little more relaxed, and a little more comfortable.

MENTAL PRACTICE AND IMAGERY IN RELAXATION

Mental practice is a symbolized rehearsal of a physical activity in the absence of any gross muscular movement. This means that a person imagines in his or her own mind the way to perform a given activity. *Imagery* is concerned with the development of a mental image that may aid one in the performance of an activity. In mental practice, the person thinks through what is going to be done, and with imagery he or she may suggest (or another may suggest a condition) and he or she then tries to effect a mental image of the condition.

The use of mental practice in performing motor skills is not new. In fact, research in this general area has been going on for well over half a century. This research has revealed that imagining a movement will likely produce recordable electric action potentials emanating from the muscles groups that would be called up if the movement were to be actually carried out. In addition, most mental activity is accompanied by a general rise in muscular tension.

One procedure in the use of mental practice for relaxation is that of making suggestions to one's self. For the most part, in early childhood, we first learn to act on the basis of verbal instructions from others. Later we learn to guide and direct our own behavior on the basis of our own language activities—we literally talk to ourselves, giving ourselves instructions. This point of view has long been supported by research that postulates that speech as a form of communication between children and adults later becomes a means of organizing the child's own behavior.

That is, the function that was previously divided between two people—child and adult—becomes an internal function of human behavior.

One way imagery can be used to promote a relaxed state is by making short comparative statements to children such as "float like a feather" or "melt like ice."

Two of my collaborators on a writing project, the previously mentioned John Carter and Harold Russel, have prepared a tape called "Float Ride" which focuses on visual imagery. The following narrative is presented in a soft, slow, and soothing voice, giving children plenty of time to listen, absorb, and passively follow the directions. The dashes represent pauses. Soft music is in the background.

FLOAT RIDE

Now, get in a very comfortable position—
Close your eyes and try to relax your body—
Think about your breathing—
Breathe in—Breathe out—
Breathe in through your nose and out through your mouth—
Now take a deep breath, hold it—
Let it out slowly—
Feel yourself sinking deeper and deeper into the chair—
You're beginning to feel very comfortable and relaxed—
Today we're going to take a ride on a float in the Gulf. We each have a float and it needs to be blown up—
So first thing we do is blow them up. Take your float and blow into it, by taking deep breaths and exhaling into the float—
You will need to blow up your float at least ten times—
So now, take a very deep breath and, slowly exhale into your float—
Each time you breathe out, let your body become more and more relaxed—
Each breath should let you feel good inside—
Now that our floats are blown up, we'll walk down to the water—
The sun is very bright and it feels warm on your skin—
The sand feels warm and cushy and soft against your feet—
As we get closer to the water we can smell the salty air—
We can hear the waves—of the ocean as they hit the beach—
The water is closer now and the sand begins to get a little cooler—
The sun is shining on us and we feel good—

We will pause for a few moments now to feel the sun and the sand beneath our feet—

We are now at the edge of the water and we get on our floats—

The floats feel very comfortable and secure—

The air is warm and the water is cool—

We are slowly floating away from the shore on our floats and we feel very relaxed—

There are seagulls in the sky and we open our eyes to watch them fly by us—

The water is warm and we feel it with our hands and our legs—

The water is moving our floats away from the beach and we feel very comfortable and safe—

As the waves pass under us, the floats move slowly up, and slowly down—

We move with the floats—up, and down—up, and down—up and down very slowly—

We feel as if we were being rocked to sleep—

The water is pushing us up and down—up, and down—

We feel very relaxed and comfortable—

As the waves are passing under us, they begin to pull us closer and closer and closer to the beach—

For just a few more seconds we can ride on our float without having to touch the sand—

The sun is warming our bodies, and the float ride is relaxing our bodies and minds—

The floats touch the sand and we must get our bodies to move again—

So for a few seconds, bring yourself back to alertness and get off the float—

The sand feels warm against our feet once more and we feel very good inside and outside—

The air is warm and is drying our bodies quickly as we slowly walk away from the water—

Now we let the air out of our floats, and with each gust of wind escaping from the float we let it relax our bodies—

Now we have finished with the ride and with the floats and must return to the room—

As I count backward from five to one, slowly bring yourself back to being alert and relaxed—

5—

4—Begin to feel more alert and allow energy to come into your body—
3—Move your arms and legs—
2—Wiggle your fingers and your toes—open your eyes
1—Sit up, stretch and feel alert and good all over.

A child stress management specialist who has had much success in using imagery to help children relax is Gretchen Koehler.[8] She has developed a number of routines for this purpose, some examples of which follow:

1. Take a walk in nature. Choose areas from soothing greens and cool blues. View distant objects, and also look closely at nature. Have your students lie on the grass and listen to natural sounds.
2. While sitting or lying down, imagine the warmth of the sun on your shoulders, arms, hands, legs, your whole body. Repeat phrases like "Think about your hands; can you make them feel warm and heavy?" Teach the children to say to themselves, "I feel warm all over. I am calm and warm."
3. Count to ten aloud slowly while your students relax. Have them concentrate on slow breathing as they visualize the numbers. When the number ten is reached, the routine is over and students open their eyes and stretch.
4. Use of nature sounds has a relaxing effect on children. Play a tape of such sounds as birds, wind, ocean waves, or rain. Instruct your students to listen and picture the place where they might hear these sounds.
5. Use quiet words to describe things that children can identify with and ask them to visualize as you speak. "Can you see a beautiful flower in your mind?" "Can you see a mountain or beach"?
6. Instruct your students to quietly repeat calm statements after you have said them. For instance, "I am calm;" "I am quiet;" "I feel relaxed."

In closing this section of the chapter, a word of caution is submitted. Although mental practice and imagery are sound techniques for helping children relax, it is possible that certain children could have side effects. For example, a borderline psychotic child could possibly be harmed by imagery activities.

---
8 Koehler, Gretchen. Stress Management for Children. *Strategies*, November/December, 1987.

HELPING CHILDREN LEARN ABOUT REST, SLEEP, AND RELAXATION

For effective learning, concepts related to rest, sleep, and relaxation can be integrated successfully with other areas of emphasis, such as (1) rest before and after meals, (2) rest and digestion, (3) balance of exercise and rest, (4) rest and body functions, (5) rest in the prevention and cure of diseases, and (6) rest and emotional health. The emphasis at the kindergarten and primary levels is on the development of practices regarding regular hours of sleep and ways of resting, and relaxing. Fourth-grade children learn about the *value* of sleep. At the fifth-grade level the emphasis is on sleep and *body growth and development.* Sixth-grade content deals with sleep and *bodily function.* Following are some suggested concepts that might be developed.

Kindergarten

We rest after we play.
We rest when we are tired.
Story time is a quiet, restful time.

Grade 1

We grow when we sleep.
Regular hours for going to bed and for getting up help us get the sleep we need.
A bath before bedtime can help us sleep better.

Grade 2

To prepare for sleep it is helpful to take a bath and clean our teeth.
Rest before dinner can help us to enjoy our meal.
Listening to a story or to music is a good way to relax after play.
Lack of sleep can make us irritable, tired, and quarrelsome.

Grade 3

Our bodies need a balance between rest and exercise.
Relaxing activities before bedtime can help us to sleep well.

Sleep helps the body get ready for the next day's work or play.
A regular amount of sleep every night can make us lively and happy.

Grade 4

Sufficient sleep aids growth, stimulates alertness, and can improve our disposition.
A warm bath or shower at bedtime is a good way to relax.
Balance between work and play activities can help to prevent fatigue.
Sleep helps our bodies build defense against disease.
Sleep is a time well suited for the body to grow.

Grade 5

Regular sleeping hours are important to healthful living.
Sleep and rest give the body a chance to rebuild cells and get rid of waste.
Sleep and rest are important to improve the strength of muscles.
Sleep relaxes tired nerves.
Rest aids digestion.
Sleep and rest are an aid to proper body mechanics.

Grade 6

Sleep is a basic need which helps the body function properly.
During sleep the circulatory system carries off the waste stored in muscle tissues.
During sleep the body refreshes itself as the processes slow down.
Sleep gives rest to the nerve cells.
Rest in bed when ill helps the white blood cells fight germs.
Doing things that interest us help us to relax.

Chapter 7

STRESS AND CHILD HEALTH

Although we tend to think of stress as being mainly concerned with the adult population, there is plenty of evidence to demonstrate that it can have a devastating effect on growing children. There is no question about it, stress can take a tremendous toll on the physical, social, and emotional health of children. It is the purpose of this chapter to discuss various aspects of childhood stress that can impact upon the health of children.

It is interesting to note that many persons believe stress in children does not begin to be important until after a child is able to walk and talk. However, there is no question that before this stage of development many children will be victims of some sort of stress. In fact, it is now known that fetuses respond to maternal stress and that newborns may respond to stress that develops in their parents owing to failure of the newborn to grow, or to colick in the newborn.

It is the general belief that infants are unaware of the differences between self and physical and human environments. Many child development specialists feel that the two most important tasks of the infant and the child up to about age two are to establish inner images of the outer world of people and objects. In the process of establishing such images, life can be unpleasant for this age cohort and, as a result, they may become stressed. In this regard, the following two studies are of interest.

In one study Szur[1] discusses the awareness of the continuities in the meaning of relationships from the beginning of life that forms the basis of the work that has been carried out by a number of psychoanalysts and child psychotherapists in infant intensive care units. Observations of mothers and babies formed the core and common starting point of the work. Newborns take an interest in people before objects; their senses

---

1 Szur, Rolene, Hospital Care of the Newborn: Some Aspects of Personal Stress, Introduction: Infants in Hospitals, *Journal of Child Psychotherapy*, 7(2), 1981.

enable them to distinguish their mother's smell, voice and face within the first few days and weeks. In a neonatal unit or labor ward, the interaction between parents, professionals and the institution presents stresses and difficulties. It is suggested that the baby in intensive care may not have small needs answered because the meaningful details in context and sequence that give clues to his or her experience are not observed. Two case studies of a 14-week-old male whose needs were met and a newborn male with a tracheostomy whose needs were not met are given as examples. It was suggested that although family presence for child patients is important, unless the staff is sensitive and understanding, there is a risk of placing too much emphasis on this aspect.

In the second study Earnshaw[2] reports on an observation made in a special-care baby unit, that rectal temperature-taking often changed the babies' respiration, general movement, facial expression, and color. Changes were most marked in the newest and smallest babies as respiration diminished, general movement slowed, and the baby took on a vacant facial expression. It was suggested that newborns express their needs in physical ways, and that caretakers must develop capacities to observe without preconceptions, but with attentiveness and openness.

As children begin the various stages of development, many are beset with problems of stress. The very first stage of child development, the period from birth to about 15 months, is considered to be the "intake" stage, because behavior and growth are characterized by *taking in*. This not only applies to food but to other things, such as sound, light, and the various forms of total care. At this early stage of the child's life *separation anxiety* can begin. Since the child is entirely dependent on the mother or other caregiver to meet its needs, separation may be seen as being deprived of these important needs. It is at this stage that the child's overseer—ordinarily the parent—should try to maintain a proper balance between meeting the child's needs and "overgratification." Many child development experts seem to agree that children who experience some stress from separation or from having to wait for a need to be fulfilled are gaining the opportunity to organize their psychological resources and to adapt to stress. On the contrary, children who did not have this balance may tend to disorganize under stress.

During the stage from about 15 months to three years, children are

---

[2] Earnshaw, A. Hospital Care of the Newborn: Some Aspects of Personal Stress: Action Consultancy. *Journal of Child Psychotherapy* 7(2), 1981.

said to develop autonomy. This can be described as the "I am what I can do" stage. Autonomy develops because most children can now move about rather easily. The child does not have to rely entirely on a caregiver to meet every single need. Autonomy also results from the development of mental processes, because the child can think about things and put language to use.

It is during this stage that the process of toilet training can be a major stressor. Children are not always given the needed opportunity to express autonomy during this process. It can be a difficult time for the child, because he or she is ordinarily expected to cooperate with, and gain the approval of, the principal caregiver. If the child cooperates and uses the toilet, approval is forthcoming; however, some autonomy is lost. If the child does not cooperate, disapproval may result. If this conflict is not resolved satisfactorily, some clinical psychologists believe it will emerge during adulthood in the form of highly anxious and compulsive behaviors.

The next stage from three to five years, can be described as "I am what I think I am." Children develop the ability to daydream and make believe, and these are used to manifest some of their behaviors. Pretending allows them to be what they want to be—anything from astronauts to zebras. It is possible, however, that resorting to too much fantasy may result in stress, because the children may become scared of their own fantasies.

Unquestionably children at all early age levels, beginning at birth (and possibly before as well) are likely to encounter a considerable amount of stress in our complex modern society. The objectives of parents and teachers should be to help them to reduce distress by making a change in the environment and/or making a change in the children themselves.

The child's various environments abound with many stress-inducing factors. The two most prominent of these environments are the home and school environments. For nine months of the year the home and school environments occupy practically all of the time of children in the age range from 6 to 12. Specifically, children spend about two-thirds of their waking hours in the home environment and the remaining one-third in the school environment. Later in the chapter we will examine certain aspects of these two environments that induce stress in children. Such information should be useful to parents and teachers by helping them to become more aware of these factors and at the same time assisting children to deal with them. Before that, however, let us consider the subject of *stress* itself.

THE MEANING OF STRESS

There is no solid agreement regarding the derivation of the term *stress*. Some sources suggest that the term is derived from the Latin word *stringere* meaning to "bind tightly." Other sources contend that the term derives from the French word *destress* (English—*distress*) and suggest that the prefix "dis" was eventually eliminated because of slurring, as in the case of the word *because* sometimes becoming *'cause*.

A common generalized literal description of the term is a "constraining force or influence." When applied to human beings, this could be interpreted to mean the extent to which the body can withstand a given force or influence. In this regard one of the most often quoted descriptions of stress is that of the late Hans Selye, who described it as the "nonspecific response of the body to any demand made upon it." Dr. Selye, one of the most renowned scientists of modern times, has generally been referred to as the "Father of Stress." It was my good fortune to collaborate with him on certain aspects of childhood stress in the late 1970s.

Selye's definition means that stress involves a mobilization of the bodily resources to some sort of stimulus (stressor). These responses can include various physical and chemical changes in the body. This description of stress could be extended by saying that it involves demands that tax and/or exceed the resources of the human body. This means that stress not only involves these bodily responses, but it also involves wear and tear on the body brought about by these responses. In essence, stress can be considered as any factor acting internally or externally that makes it difficult to adapt and that induces increased effort on the part of a person to maintain a state of balance within himself and with his external environment. It should be understood that stress is a *state* that one is in, and this should not be confused with any stimuli that produces such a state (stressors).

THE CONCEPT OF STRESS

In discussing the stress concept I do not intend to get into a highly technical discourse on the complex and complicated aspect of stress.

Nonetheless, there are certain basic understandings that need to be taken into account, and this requires the use of some technical terms. For this reason I am providing a "minidictionary" of terms used in the discussion to follow.

> ACTH—(*A*dreno*C*ortico*T*ropic*H*ormone) secreted by the pituitary gland. It influences the function of the adrenals and other glands in the body.
>
> ADRENALIN—A hormone secreted by the medulla of the adrenal glands.
>
> ADRENALS—Two glands in the upper posterior part of the abdomen that produce and secrete hormones. They have two parts, the outer layer, called the *cortex* and the inner core called the *medulla.*
>
> CORTICOIDS—Hormones produced by the adrenal cortex, an example of which is *cortisone.*
>
> ENDOCRINE—Glands that secrete their hormones into the blood stream.
>
> HORMONE—A chemical produced by a gland, secreted into the blood stream, and influencing the function of cells or organs.
>
> HYPOTHALAMUS—The primary activator of the autonomic nervous system, it plays a central role in translating neurological stimuli into endocrine processes during stress reactions.
>
> PITUITARY—An endocrine gland located at the base of the brain about the size of a pea. It secretes important hormones, one of which is the ACTH hormone.
>
> THYMUS—A ductless gland that is considered a part of the endocrine gland system, located behind the upper part of the breast bone.

Although there are various theories of stress, one of the basic and better known ones is that of the previously-mentioned Hans Selye. I have already given Selye's description of stress as the "nonspecific response of the body to any demand made upon it." The physiological processes and reactions involved in Selye's stress model is identified as the *General Adaptation Syndrome* and consists of the three stages of *alarm reaction, resistance stage,* and the *exhaustion stage.*

In the first stage (alarm reaction), the body reacts to the stressor and causes the hypothalamus to produce a biochemical "messenger," which in turn causes the pituitary gland to secrete ACTH into the blood. This hormone then causes the adrenal gland to discharge adrenalin and other corticoids. This causes shrinkage of the thymus with an influence on heart rate, blood pressure and the like. It is during the alarm stage that the resistance of the body is reduced.

In the second stage, *resistance* develops if the stressor is not too pronounced. Body adaptation develops to fight back the stress or possibly avoid it, and the body begins to repair damage, if any.

The third stage of *exhaustion* occurs if there is long-continued exposure to the same stressor. The ability of adaptation is eventually exhausted and the signs of the first stage (alarm reaction) reappear. Selye contended that our adaptation resources are limited, and when they become irreversible, the result is death. The goal of all of us, of course, should be to keep our resistance and capacity for adaptation.

Although Selye's stress model which places emphasis upon "nonspecific" responses has been widely accepted, in recent years the nonspecific nature of stress has been questioned by some. Some findings tend to support the idea that there are other hormones involved in stress in addition to those of the pituitary-adrenal system.

As in the case of all scientific research, the search for truth continues and more sophisticated procedures will emerge in the study of stress, and current theories will be more critically appraised. In the meantime, there is abundant evidence to support the notion that stress in modern society is a serious threat to the well-being of man if not controlled, and of course, the most important factor in such control is man himself.

HOME AND FAMILY STRESS

The magnitude of home and family stress is well-documented. For example, in Coddington's[3] list of the 36 life events that are most stressful for children, well over one-half of them are concerned with home and family. Without question changes in society with consequent changes in conditions in some homes are likely to make child adjustment a difficult problem.

Such factors as changes in standards of female behavior, larger percentages of both parents working, economic conditions, mass media such as television, as well as numerous others can complicate the life of the modern-day child.

---

[3] Coddington, R. D., Measuring the Stressfulness of a Child's Environment, In *Stress in Childhood*, Edited by James H. Humphrey, New York, AMS Press, Inc., 1984.

Specific research studies tend to focus on a more or less single aspect of home and family stress. Representative examples are presented here in the categories of (1) child abuse, (2) divorce and marital dissolution, and (3) life changes. It should be understood that there is likely to be some overlapping from one of these categories to another.

Child Abuse

It is estimated that one million or more children are abused or neglected by their parents or other "overseers" in our country annually, and that as many as 2,000 die as a result of maltreatment. Authorities suggest that much of this is not caused by inhuman, hateful intent on the part of parents, but rather it is the result of a combination of factors including both the accumulation of stresses on families and unmet needs of parents for support in coping with their child bearing responsibilities.

There are various ways in which stress is related to child abuse. Some examples of this type of research are presented in the following discussion.

An attempt to provide an integrative framework for understanding child maltreatment was undertaken by Pianta.[4] He drew on data collected as a part of the Mother-Child Interaction Project at the University of Minnesota, which involved a longitudinal study of 267 primiparous women (and their children) considered at risk for child abuse, to provide an integrative framework for understanding child maltreatment. The subjects were identified on the basis of referrals to child protection agencies and matched with groups of nonabusing and excellent-care parents from the same sample. Comparisons of mothers in the two groups showed that abusing mothers were of lower intelligence and had negative reactions, expectations, and low self-images. Although irritability of children has been associated with child abuse, the quality of the maternal response determines the quality of the relationship. Social stressors associated with child abuse include unemployment, lack of social support, stressful life events, and high levels of confusion. It was suggested that sociological and maternal characteristics are inextricably intertwined in mutual cause relationships in child abuse. Early separation during the pripartum period (failure of bond formation) has also

---

[4] Pianta, B., Antecedents of Child Abuse: Single and Multiple Factors Models, *Minneapolis School Psychology Interaction Project*, 5.

been associated with abuse and neglect of mothers. Pianta concluded that treatment and prevention must address a combination of variables.

In a similar type of study Howze and Kotch[5] investigated the potential for child abuse and neglect. They suggested that although there is a growing body of literature linking stress to child abuse and neglect, the relationship is not unambiguously supported by empirical data. They believe that two considerations regarding an ecological model of child abuse and neglect may explain this research problem. First, predisposing factors (which are grouped into four levels called individual, familial, social, and cultural) may either positively or negatively affect the potential for child abuse and neglect, depending on the quality of social networks and social support available to families. Second, these factors operate most importantly, not between the perception of stress and the act of abuse or neglect, but through the interpretation of whether a given life event is stressful or not. This clarification of the ecological model points the way to redefining interventions for the primary prevention of child abuse and neglect. Existing support systems can be strengthened in order to increase a family's ability to cope with untoward events before these become stressful. In addition, advocacy activities that support children and families in general can be major components in the primary prevention of child abuse and neglect.

Gaudin and Pollane[6] investigated the relationship between situational stress of informal social networks, and maternal child abuse. Structured interviews were conducted with 41 abusive mothers and 59 nonabusing mothers using an instrument developed by the researchers to measure social network strength and situational stress. Abusing mothers, on the average, reported significantly weaker, less supportive informal social networks than the nonabusing mothers. Both the neighbor/friend networks and the kinship networks of the nonabusing mothers were found to be stronger than those of abusing mothers. The data also supported the positive association of situational stress with child abuse. Both situational stress and strength of social support proved to be significant predictors of abuse. The findings supported the hypothesized effect of strong social networks upon the relationship between situational stress and child abuse. Mothers living in highly stressful life situations who

---
5 Howze, D. C. and Kotch, J. B., Disentangling Life Events and Social Support: Implications for the Primary Prevention of Child Abuse and Neglect, *Child Abuse and Neglect*, 8.
6 Gaudin, J. M. and Pollane, L., *Children and Youth Services Review*, 5, 1984.

reported strong social networks were less likely to be abusers than mothers living in high-stress situations who reported weak social networks. The mediating functions of social networks were proposed, and the implications of the findings for interventions with high-risk parents to prevent child abuse were deemed important.

The final study involving stress and child abuse reported here is one in which Mash, Johnston and Kovitch[7] made a comparison of the mother-child interactions of physically abused and nonabused children during play and task situations. They observed 18 physically abusive mothers (AMs) and their 18 children (mean age 55.44 months) and 18 nonabusive mothers (NAMs) and their 18 children matched for age, sex, and IQ to children of the AMs interacting in both unstructured play and a structured task situation. Mothers also completed several checklists describing their children and themselves. Results indicated that AMs perceived their children as having significantly more behavioral problems than did NAMs. AMs were observed to be more directive and controlling of their children, but only for the more stressful situations in which there were increased demands for performance placed on both mother and child. AMs reported higher levels of stress related to parenting than NAMs; these reports were correlated with their behavior both during the play and task situations. The findings indicated that in AMs there was failure to regulate their behavior in relation to the performance of their children and the possibility that such a response style is more likely to occur in the context of situationally-induced stress.

Divorce and Marital Dissolution

During the past 25 years, the number of children who have experienced parental divorce has tripled. In the 1990s it is expected that almost one-half of all children will have experienced parental divorce during childhood or adolescence.

Depression, anger, self-blame, anxiety, and low self-esteem frequently occur after divorce. In addition to social interaction problems, noncompliance, aggression, and school difficulties occur more frequently among children of divorce than children from impact families. For some children,

---

[7] Mash, E. J., Johnston, C., and Kovitch, K. A., A Comparison of the Mother-Child Interaction of Physically Abused and Nonabused Children During Play and Task Situations, *Journal of Clinical Child Psychology*, 12, 1983.

divorce produces mild or transient behavior problems, but for many others, this transition in family structure leads to enduring emotional and behavioral difficulties.

Hetherington,[8] approaching it from a child's perspective contended that much of the confusion in studying the impact of divorce on children has been a result of failure to view divorce as a process involving a series of events and changes in life circumstance rather than as a single event. At different points in this sequence children are confronted with different adaptive tasks and will use different coping strategies. The diversity in children's responses to divorce in part is attributable to temperamental status. In understanding the child's adjustment to divorce it is important to look not only at changes in family structure but also at changes in family functioning and at stresses and support systems in the child's extrafamilial social environment.

In another study Woody[9] examined child adjustment to parental stress following divorce. She studied the relationship of parental stress and adjustment to child adjustment in 87 parents (most of whom were aged 24-35 years) who were either divorced or divorcing and their 181 children (aged 1-17 years). Parents were administered demographic, parent and child mental health, life stress, parental communication and contact, and current family relationship measures. It was found that high levels of parent stress, parent symptomatology, and a spouse-type relationship predict greater numbers of child symptoms that do not decrease with passing of time. Moreover, younger parents and those who used little help or felt that the help used was not valuable reported more child symptoms. These findings mandate a strong child advocacy role for helping professionals that consist of the development and delivery of prevention programs and the use of directive psychoeducational approaches in clinical practice.

In the final study of divorce and marital dissolution reported here Cohen[10] investigated the impact of marital dissolution on personal distress and childrearing attitudes of mothers. She examined the impact of separation and divorce on 79 25 to 48-year-old mothers of one or more 4 to 12-year-old children. She administered an adjustment inventory and

---

8 Hetherington, E., Divorce, a Child's Perspective, *Annual Progress in Child Psychiatry and Child Development.* 1980.

9 Woody, J. D., Child Adjustment to Parental Stress Following Divorce, *Social Casework*, 65, 1984.

10 Cohen, J., The Impact of Marital Dissolution on Personal Distress and Childrearing Attitudes of Mothers, *Journal of Orthomolecular Psychiatry*, 2, 1983.

a parent attitude survey to the subjects and to 52 matched and married mothers. The results showed that personal distress and childrearing attitudes were rarely influenced by age, number of children, or length of marriage. Married subjects showed significantly lower indices of personal distress. It was suggested that the personal experience of turmoil may be attributed to the demands of single parenthood, even though 74 percent of separated subjects felt they had a more satisfying lifestyle after divorce.

Life Changes

Although some children seem to take any kind of change in their lives in stride, many others tend to suffer serious distress as a result of it. Oftentimes there can be certain psychological consequences because of life changes.

Stewart and her associates[11] studied this phenomenon by conducting several longitudinal studies of children and adults to assess the validity of a hypothesized process of internal adaptation to external life changes. Data on the Thematic Apperception Test (TAT) were collected twice over three years from 284 students entering junior high school, 55 children in kindergarten through second grade, 113 students entering college, and 94 adults beginning marriage or becoming parents. It was hypothesized that changes would precipitate a receptive, dependent stance toward external environment and that the postchange period would be characterized by gradual adoption of more assertive, or integrated stances. Results supported the hypotheses and indicated that additional changes in the posttraction period may interfere with adaptation to the initial change. There was evidence that males and females may differ in their tolerance of the receptive and assertive stances.

In a study involving family relocation, Gullotta and Donohue[12] examined the effects that moving and separation have on families and suggested a role for mental health agencies in easing these stressful life events. Knowledge of family separation, father's entry and reentry into the family, and mobility in general originates from studies of military families showing that those best able to adapt to the frequent arrivals and

---

11 Stewart, A. J., et al. Longitudinal Studies of Psychological Consequences of Life Change in Children and Adults. *Journal of Personality and Social Psychology*, 50, 1986.

12 Gullotta, T. P. and Donohue, K. C., Families, Relocation, and the Corporation, *New Directions for Mental Health Services*, 20, 1983.

departures experience low levels of rootlessness. Families that experience heightened alienation experience greater problems. Children whose fathers are frequently absent are reported to experience greater dependency needs and more academic problems and to have higher referral rates for emotional problems. Literature on stress in the corporate family parallels findings on military families. A move consists of four stages: (1) preparation, (2) migration, (3) overcompensation, and (4) decompensation. Approaches used to strengthen family functioning during relocation include: (1) education, (2) competency promotion, (3) community organization, and (4) natural caregiving. Four factors of corporation assistance are recommended and include the establishment of relocation officers to oversee operations, a site visit by the family, educational seminars for employees and spouses, and publications about moving. It was concluded that community care and information can ease the stress of moving families and help them to cope with new circumstances.

SCHOOL STRESS

In Coddington's previously-mentioned list of 36 life events, over 10% of them are concerned with the school environment and they are highly weighted as being stressful for children. Indeed, there are a number of conditions existing in many school situations that can cause much stress for children and thus impact on child health. These conditions prevail at all levels—possibly in different ways—from the time a child enters school until graduation from college.

Thoresen and Eagleston[13] have discussed the consequences of experiencing prolonged chronic stress for students in the education system, from preschool to graduate school. They believe that the child or adolescent who is facing a set of demands with insufficient resources may respond in many ways that are harmful or maladaptive.

Miscoping responses can include behavioral and environmental responses such as social withdrawal, alcohol or drug abuse, and truancy. In the cognitive area, an imbalance of demands and resources could result in feelings of low self-esteem and beliefs about being a failure. Related to these is the possible evolution of "learned helplessness," the belief that one's actions essentially are unrelated to the consequences that are

---

13 Thoresen, C. E. and Eagleston, J. R., Chronic Stress in Children and Adolescents, *Theory into Practice*, 22, 1983.

experienced. Strategies for overcoming chronic stress, such as physical exercise and the learning of new social skills, are highly recommended by these authors.

Stress and the Child in the Educative Process

School anxiety as a child stressor is a phenomenon with which educators, particular teachers and counselors, frequently find themselves confronted in dealing with children. Various theories have been advanced to explain this phenomenon and relate it to other character traits and emotional dispositions. Literature on the subject reveals the following characteristics of anxiety as a stress inducing factor in the educative process.

1. Anxiety is considered a learnable reaction that has the properties of a response, a cue of danger, and a drive.
2. Anxiety is internalized fear aroused by the memory of painful past experiences associated with punishment for the gratification of an impulse.
3. Anxiety in the classroom interferes with learning and whatever can be done to reduce it should serve as a spur to learning.
4. Test anxiety is a near universal experience, especially in this country, which is a test-giving and test-conscious culture.
5. Evidence from clinical studies points clearly and consistently to the disruption and distracting power of anxiety effects over most kinds of thinking.

It would seem that causes of anxiety change with age as do perceptions of stressful situations. Care should be taken in assessing the total life space of the child—background, home life, school life, age, and sex—in order to minimize the anxiety experienced in the school. It seems obvious that school anxiety, although manifested in the school environment, may often be caused by unrelated factors outside the school.

Conners[14] studied certain interactions with the educative process as they relate to stress. He discussed growing evidence that the designed environment of schools may stress users of the facility both directly and indirectly. Several areas where the designed environment, both on a school-wide and classroom level, interacts with the educational process were explored, and these interactions were considered from the perspec-

---

14 Conners, D. A., The School Environment: A Link to Understanding Stress, *Theory into Practice*, 22, 1983.

tive of stresses imposed on both teacher and student. Seating position, classroom design and arrangement, density and crowding, privacy, and noise were considered. He suggests that schools need to provide places that will enhance goals for interaction, for participation in social networks, and for control over the time and place for social interactions. Relatively minor design modifications introduced into already functioning classrooms have been shown to produce changes in students' spatial behavior, increased interaction with materials, and decreased interruptions.

Obviously cognitive behaviors are important in the educative process and for success in school. In this regard Houston, Fox and Forbes[15] studied this factor as it was concerned with children's state anxiety and performance under stress. They evaluated the relations between trait anxiety in children and state anxiety, cognitive behaviors, and performance in a single study in which two levels of stress were experimentally manipulated.

Sixty-seven 4th grade children (41 females, 26 males) anticipated and then performed a mathematics task in either a high- or low-stress condition. While the children anticipated performing the task, measures of seven cognitive behaviors were obtained by means of a think-aloud procedure and a cognitive behavior questionnaire. The children were also administered the State-Trait Anxiety Inventory for Children. Trait anxiety was found to be related to state anxiety and the cognitive behaviors of preoccupation, and for females, justification of positive attitudes. The performance of high but not low-anxious children was affected by levels of success. This finding aids in reconciling discrepancies in previous research concerning children's trait anxiety and performance.

If the child is to be successful in the educative process and to achieve, it is imperative that he or she be able to make the best use of native intelligence. The fact that stress can have a negative impact on IQ and task performance is shown in the work of Bernard Brown and Lilian Rosenbaum,[16] two eminent researchers on the subject, and collaborators of mine on a stress project. The following discussion consists of some of the excerpted materials of their work in this field.

They examined the effects of stress on IQ in a sample of 4,154 of 41,540 seven-year-old children from the Collaborative Project. They developed a stress index which was a composite score of the number of medical/

---

[15] Houston, B., Fox, J. E., and Forbes, L., Trait Anxiety and Children's State Anxiety, Cognitive Behaviors, and Performance Under Stress, *Cognitive Therapy and Research*, 8, 1984.

[16] Brown, Bernard B. and Rosenbaum, Lilian, Stress and Competence, In *Stress in Childhood*, Edited by James H. Humphrey, New York, AMS Press, Inc., 1984.

psychological problems found in a child. The variables were selected from the Collaborative Project data files collected in the 1960s. They included mother's marital status, employment, family configuration, history of illness, death, and divorce in the family, measures of autonomic function, achievement measures, and physician-identified health disorders including vision, motor, speech, and hearing problems. They found an inverted-U curve of performance on the WISC IQ test and its component subtests for IQ vs. stress level as measured by total number of problems per child. For example, on the WISC Information subtest white, middle-class children with three problems scored the equivalent of eight IQ points higher than those with no problems and 13 points higher than those with ten problems. The Information, Block Design, and Coding subtests have the greatest sensitivity to stress and the Comprehension and Vocabulary subtests were the least sensitive. The inverted-U curve of the full-scale WISC IQ test was less pronounced than the curves of the subtests with only a seven-point difference between maximum performance level and the performance level under high stress. The curves of low SES children were of the same inverted-U form but were peaked at lower stress levels suggesting higher arousal and stressor levels. Thus, the researchers showed that stress has a large effect on intelligence test scores.

On the basis of their work and a review of the literature they have put forward a body of evidence to support the hypothesis that stress affects intelligence. They presented evidence that many families are exposed to high stressor levels, both acute and chronic. Stress affects the level of anxiety, sense of mastery, self-esteem, depression, and general ability to function in the family which in turn shapes children's competence. Stressors influence performance both immediately and developmentally as they interact with genetics, environment, and experience to shape physical, social, emotional, and intellectual growth.

They have also presented evidence that acute stressors disrupt the balance between cognitive and emotional function as highly differentiated thought decreases and the brain becomes emotionally overreactive. Children who experience chronic stressors, either real or perceived, show long-term decline in intelligence if their coping skills are inadequate, while children with appropriate skills rise in intelligence.

They suggest that the hypothesis that stress affects competence implies a different set of interactions in dealing with dysfunction in children and families. Competence in functioning can be altered by modifying the degree of individual differentiation, the intensity, frequency, and predictability of the stressors, and/or the individual's response (arousal) to the stressors and processes of family function. These interpretations can alter the present competence of the individual as well as presumably counter the transmission of suboptimal functioning across generations. These include education in family processes and/or therapy as well as training in a variety of self-regulation techniques such as biofeedback and stress management. There are ways to increase the number of stress resisting factors to protect children from unnecessary risk. There can be intervention in schools and other organizations to insure that organizational processes do not lead to overreactivity in children and families.

School Subjects as Stressors

There are various subject areas that could be considered as perennial nemeses for many students. Probably any subject could be stress inducing for certain students. Prominent among those subjects that have a reputation for being more stress inducing than others are those concerned with the 3Rs. For example, it has been reported that for many children, attending school daily and performing poorly is a source of considerable and prolonged stress. If children overreact to environmental stresses in terms of increased muscle tension, this may interfere easily with the fluid muscular movement required in handwriting tasks, decreasing their performance and further increasing environmental stresses. Many educators have seen children squeeze their pencils tightly, press hard on their paper, purse their lips, and tighten their bodies, using an inordinate amount of energy and concentration to write while performing at a very low level.[17]

Reading is another area of school activity that is loaded with anxiety, stress, and frustration for many children. In fact, one of the levels of reading recognized by reading specialists is called the "frustration level." In terms of behavioral observations this can be described as the level in which children evidence tension, excessive or erratic body movement, nervousness, and distractibility. This frustration level is said to be a sign of emotional tension or stress with breakdowns in fluency and significant increase in reading errors.

---

17 Carter, J. L. and Russell, H. L., Relationship Between Reading Frustration and Muscle Tension in Children with Reading Disabilities, *American Journal of Clinical Feedback*, 2, 1979.

A study by Swain[18] was undertaken to determine the extent to which stress was a factor in primary school children's reading difficulties. She investigated referral and evaluation statements and diagnostic data from parents, teachers, reading specialists, and counselors regarding signs of stress and potential stressors as factors in the reading difficulties of 77 primary school children referred for evaluation at the Pupil Appraisal Center (PAC) at North Texas State University between 1977 and 1984.

Qualitative methods, specifically, situational analysis, were employed to obtain a holistic view of each child's reading difficulties. The researcher collected data from documented files at PAC. Data analysis via a categorical coding system produced 39 stress-related categories, organized under broad headings of family and school environment, readiness for reading/learning, general stress reactions, and responses to stress when reading/learning becomes a problem.

The most significant signs of stress cited in this study were symptoms of anxiety and a marked tendency toward passivity and unassertiveness. Primary potential stressors also emerged. Intellectual and language deficits were noted, along with self-defeating behaviors, absence of self-motivating/self-control, and problems stemming from the home and school environments.

Support for findings in referral and evaluation statements was found in diagnostic data which included intelligence, reading, and projective tests. Some of the children had specific personal limitations that might have hindered reading. However, many were experiencing frustration from working at capacity and yet not meeting parental or teacher expectations. No child was found to be coping effectively with apparent adverse circumstances. Failure by many of these children to adapt successfully to stress in their personal lives could forecast chronic difficulty in reading when it, too, becomes a challenge to them.

The subject that appears to stress the greatest majority of students is mathematics. This condition prevails from the study of arithmetic upon entering school through the required courses in mathematics in college. This has become such a problem that there is now an area of study called "Math Anxiety" that is receiving increasing attention. Prominent among those studying the phenomenon is Sheila Tobias[19] who believes that

---

18 Swain, C. J., Stress as a Factor in Primary School Children's Reading Difficulties: Some Implications for Remedial Reading, *Doctoral Dissertation*, North Texas State University, Denton, Texas, 1985.

19 Tobias, Sheila, Stress in the Math Classroom, *Learning*, January 1981.

there appears to be what could be called "math anxious" and "math avoiding" people who tend not to trust their problem-solving abilities and who experience a high level of stress when asked to use them. Even though these people are not necessarily "mathematically ignorant," they tend to feel that they are, simply because they cannot focus on the problem at hand or because they are unable to remember the appropriate formula. Thus, feelings of frustration and incompetence are likely to make them reluctant to deal with mathematics in their daily lives. It is suggested that at the root of this self-doubt is fear of making mistakes and appearing stupid in front of others.

School Tests as Stressors

At one time or another most teachers observe that many students are seriously stressed by what has become commonly known as "test anxiety."

The previously mentioned Bernard Brown and Lilian Rosenbaum contend that perceived stress appears to depend on psychological sets and responses that individuals are more likely to bring into the testing situation than manufacture on the spot. Students respond to tests and testing situations with learned patterns of stress reactivity. The patterns may vary among individuals and may reflect differences in autonomic nervous system conditioning, feelings of threat or worry regarding the symbolic meaning of the test or the testing situation, and coping skills that govern the management of complexity, frustration, information load, symbolic manipulation, and mobilization of resources. There are also individual patterns of maladaptive behavior such as anxiety, a sustained high level of automatic activity after exposure to a stressor and the use of a variety of such defense mechanisms as learned helplessness and avoidance behavior.

Parents and teachers can be of assistance to children in the rigors of test taking. Various recommendations have been made with reference as to how this can be accomplished. One qualified expert, and a collaborator of mine on a childhood stress project, Barbara Kuczen,[20] believes that the following suggestions can relieve pressure from the testing scene.

> 1. Explain the purpose of tests, and make it clear that the child's best is expected, but no more. In this way the child can prepare and

---
20 Kuczen, Barbara, *Childhood Stress Don't Let Your Child be a Victim,* New York, Delacorte Press, 1982.

relax going into the test, knowing that maximum effort is being expended.
2. When it is known that a test is scheduled, the child should get a good night's sleep, eat a well-balanced breakfast, be dressed in comfortable clothes, and leave home in a relaxed unrushed state.
3. When a test paper is returned, immediately go over the answers and analyze errors. Clear up any misunderstandings about directions, terms, or answers so the child will be better prepared the next time.
4. Give the child experience working under rigid time limits. Play some games in which the child is timed or allowed a designated number of minutes for completing a task.
5. Advise the child not to get "hung up" on a difficult question, but instead skip it and do it later, if there is time.
6. Have the child learn to pace the work by looking over the material to see how much needs to be done.
7. Have the child practice reading a question in one place and recording the answer on a separate sheet of paper.
8. Adults should not magnify the importance of tests by getting overexcited by good, or poor, scores. Let the child know that the learning that occurs in school is the prime concern. Test results should reflect that learning.
9. Help the child understand that some test stress can motivate a student to study and achieve. However, if stress is extreme, it can cripple the learner. Work on using ways to relax.
10. Help the child understand that test stress caused by not studying is likely to be inevitable and unacceptable.

Finally, it is important to take a positive attitude when considering test results. That is, emphasis should be placed on the number of answers that were correct. For example, the child will more likely be encouraged if you say, "You got seven right," rather than "You missed three." It has been my experience that this approach can help minimize stress in future test-taking.

It has been the intent of this chapter to show parents and teachers that it has been well documented that stress can have a serious impact on child health in both the home and school environments.

Chapter 8

THE ELEMENTARY SCHOOL HEALTH PROGRAM

The field of school health is characterized by the somewhat unusual distinction of having a proposed list of standardized terms. Attempts at standardization of terminology in school health began many years ago through the efforts of the Health Education Section of what was then called the American Physical Education Association. Through the years many of the health education areas took on new meanings which made it necessary to redefine terms and clarify certain features in school health. The Committee on Terminology in School Health of the American Alliance for Health, Physical Education, Recreation, and Dance has carried out this function over the years.

The terminology and definitions of the various areas of school health used here are based as far as possible upon recommendations of this committee. However, it should be borne in mind that attempts to standardize terminology in such a rapidly changing and expanding area as school health precludes a static list of standardized terms. Consequently, terminology and descriptions or definitions of the various areas of school health will deviate from the committee's recommendations as seems necessary in terms of present theories and practices.

It is a generally accepted idea that the total *school health program* involves those school procedures that contribute to the understanding, maintenance, and improvement of the health of pupils and school personnel. In carrying out these functions the total school health program is composed of three areas: *school health service, healthful school living* and *school health education.* These three areas are interrelated and, to a large extent, interdependent; they are, however, obviously separate enough to warrant individual discussions.

School Health Service

The school health service program attempts to conserve, protect, and improve the health of the school population. This objective is achieved in part through such procedures as (1) appraising the health status of pupils and school personnel; (2) counseling with pupils, parents, and others involved in the appraisal findings; (3) helping to plan for the health care and education of exceptional children; (4) helping to prevent and control disease; and (5) providing for emergency care for sick and injured pupils.

The maximum function of school health service should provide all necessary health supervision to arrive at optimal health for all children. Naturally, such service depends upon the availability of specialized personnel such as physicians, nurses, psychologists, and others who can make a worthwhile contribution to the health of children. The type and extent of service that is actually provided in a given school system also depends on such factors as available funds, size of school enrollment, and availability of properly trained personnel. Because of these factors, the range of school health services varies markedly from one school system to another.

The extreme importance of the health service aspect of the school health program is obvious when one considers the range of anomalous health conditions of the school population. For instance, some estimates indicate that, on the average, out of every one-hundred children of school age, one has heart disease, twenty have visual disorders, ten have some degree of hearing impairment, fifteen have nutritional disturbances, ten have some sort of growth problems, eighty-five have dental disease, and twenty have emotional disturbances. Added to these estimates are the facts that many children are only partially immunized, and countless others live under conditions of poor health practices that involve lack of sleep, fresh air, and sunshine.

Adequate school health services can do much to help eliminate these conditions. This is particularly true at the elementary school level because the younger the child is at the time a deviation from normal health is discovered, the greater the opportunity for proper care and possible recovery.

Role of the Classroom Teacher in School Health Service

Depending upon certain factors previously mentioned, the function of the classroom teacher in the school health service will vary from one school system to another. However, there are certain types of responsibilities that classroom teachers will likely be expected to assume in most elementary schools. Two of these major responsibilities follow.

Responsibilities concerned with health appraisal of children. Since teachers are in daily contact with children, coupled with their knowledge of growth and development, they are in an excellent position to note changes in appearance and behavior that are associated with a child's health status. When a teacher detects something that indicates a deviation from the normal health status, a referral can be made to the proper person in the health service (ordinarily the school nurse) who can follow up the referral.

Responsibility concerned with emergency illness or injury. Ideally all school personnel should have an understanding of how to care for a child in case of sudden illness or injury. It is particularly important that the classroom teacher have the skills necessary to render first aid. One of the most important factors in this regard is a teacher's full understanding of the school's policy regarding emergency care. With such knowledge at hand, the teacher can administer first aid as set forth in the prescribed school policy.

Healthful School Living

This aspect of the school health program involves procedures that provide for the most satisfactory living conditions within the school plant. Healthful school living is concerned with (1) organizing the school day on a basis commensurate with the health and safety of pupils and (2) providing for physical aspects of the school plant—proper ventilation, heating, lighting, and the other aspects that are essential for preservation of an optimum health status.

As in the case of school health service, there is likely to be a wide range of standards of healthful school living among school systems. The standard of healthful living that a given school system provides will be governed largely by available funds and specialized personnel, particularly in the area of school maintenance.

Everyone in the school system should take some degree of responsibility for ensuring satisfactory healthful school living. The position of leadership in individual schools is, of course, that of the school principal. His or her awareness of the meaning of healthful school living and how to implement it depends, to a considerable extent, upon the success of this aspect of the school health program.

Although there is no question that the principal's leadership is of prime importance to the satisfactory conducting of this environmental aspect of the school health program, the importance of other personnel should not be underestimated. Thus, classroom teachers play a major role in seeing that they and their children participate in a satisfactory manner in the program. Moreover, the teacher is in an ideal position to keep the administration sensitive to new problems and developments which require action that is beyond the teacher's scope or that of any individual class.

The children of the school, too, should be considered active participants in the maintenance of healthful school living, and, of course, the teacher can use this part of the school health program as a means of conveying basic principles of cleanliness and sanitation that are important to group living.

The role of certain other personnel in the maintenance of healthful school living is so obvious as to require only brief mention in rounding out the total picture. Physicians, nurses, custodial staff, food service personnel, and public health officers are all vitally concerned with healthful school living in the schools. Also, on occasion, problems may arise that require the attention of parent-teacher organizations as well as certain professional groups in the community.

School Health Education

It is the purpose of this aspect of the school health program to provide desirable and worthwhile learning experiences that will favorably influence knowledge, attitudes, and practices pertaining to individual and group health. The medium through which these experiences can best be provided is *health teaching*.

Without disputing the importance or even the indispensability of school health service and healthful school living, it must be emphasized that health teaching which is designed to increase the individual's ability to live healthily and deal intelligently with his or her own health problems is basic to the whole concept of healthful living. Although some efforts are being made to procure special teachers it is quite clear that the major responsibility for health teaching in the elementary school rests with the classroom teacher. However, in many situations the teacher has numerous resources to draw upon in the way of materials and various health and safety personnel connected with either the school or the local public health organization. The teacher is responsible for utilizing these in such a way that they fit into the sequence of learning experiences.

Recognition of the importance of health teaching during the early years of life has gradually resulted in a national tendency to place greater emphasis upon health in the curriculum at all grade levels. More and more schools are making a definite effort to cover a series of health topics that are considered vital to the present and future health of the child. Many states have laws requiring that certain health topics be presented. These required topics were at first quite limited, commonly amounting to the effect of alcohol, tobacco, and narcotics upon the body. However, for several years now there has been a definite trend to go far beyond teaching only those health topics required by law.

In summary, there seems to be little question that the schools have a major responsibility in promoting optimum health for children, and thus, contributing to their total development.

AFTERWORD

As mentioned in the preface, this book has been prepared for those adults—parents and teachers—who have the wherewithal to provide the guidance necessary to promote the health of children of elementary school age.

I am well aware of the fact that not all adults—particularly parents—have the necessary resources to provide for such guidance. Although it should be a foregone conclusion that the health of a child is one of the most important factors in his or her development, at the same time when one examines the comparatively low expenditures for important life values such as education and health, it becomes luminously clear that our national priorities could be subject to question as far as the welfare of our children is concerned. Many critics agree that when the federal government spends 15 times as much on the military as it does on education, there appears to be a serious distortion in the allocation of funds.

There are many deficiencies in health care in the so-called "land of plenty." Approximately 37 million Americans have no health insurance; one-third of these are children and most of the rest are the working poor. Add to this the fact that thousands upon thousands of children are members of families well below the poverty line. This number is increasing tremendously and, according to some experts, is getting out of control.

BIBLIOGRAPHY

Armstrong, N. and Davies, B., The Prevalence of Coronary Risk Factors in Children, *Acta Paediatrica Belgia,* 33, 1980.

Carson, D. K. and Greeley, S., Not by Bread Alone: Reversing the Effects of Childhood Malnutrition, *Early Child Development and Care,* 1–4, 1988.

Chandler, W. U., Child Health, Education, and Development, *Prospects,* 3, 1986.

Cureton, K., Commentary on Children and Fitness: A Public Health Perspective, *Research Quarterly for Exercise and Sports,* 58, 1987.

Garn, S. M. and LaVelle, M., Two Decade Follow-Up of Fatness in Early Childhood, *American Journal of Diseases of Children,* 138, 1985.

Giel, D., Is There a Crisis in Youth Fitness—or fatness? *Physician and Sportsmedicine,* October 1988.

Gilliam, T. B., Coronary Heart Disease Risk in Children and Their Physical Activity, In R. A. Boileau (Ed.) *Advances in Pediatric Sport Sciences,* Champaign, IL, 1984.

Gilliam, T. B., et al, Physical Activity Patterns Determined by Heart Rate Monitoring in 6–7 Year-Old Children, *Medicine and Science in Sports and Exercise,* 13, 1981.

Golebiowska, M. and Bujnowski, T., Effects of an 8-month Reducing Program on the Physical Fitness of Obese Children, In Rutenfranz J., et al, Eds.) *Children and Exercise XII,* Human Kinetics, 1986.

Gortmaker, S. L., et al, Increasing Pediatric Obesity in the *United States, American Journal of Diseases in Children,* 141, 1987.

Graham, P., Psychology and the Health of Children, *The Journal of Child Psychology and Psychiatry and Allied Disciplines,* May 1985.

Groves, D., Is Childhood Obesity Related to TV Addiction? *Physician and Sportsmedicine,* Minneapolis, November 1988.

Klesges, R. C., et al, The FATS: An Observational System for Assessing Physical Activity in Children and Associated Parental Behavior, *Behavioral Assessment,* 1983.

Lindner, E. W., Our National Health Policy of Child Carelessness, *The Education Digest,* October 1986.

McFadyen, S. C., et al, Injuries, Absences, and Visits to the Nurse Among Children in Alternative Schools, *Journal of School Health,* December 1988.

Parcel, G. S., et al, School Promotion of Healthful Diet and Exercise Behavior: An Investigation of Organization Change and Social Learning Theory Intervention, *Journal of School Health,* 57, 1987.

Parizkova, J. Growth, Functional Capacity and Physical Fitness in Normal and Malnourished Children, *World Review of Nutrition and Dietitics,* 51, 1987.

Parizkova, J., et al, Body Composition, Food Intake, Cardiorespiratory Fitness, Blood Lipids and Psychological Development in Highly Active and Inactive Preschool Children, *Human Biology,* April 1986.

Peterson L., Preventing the Leading Killer of Children: The Role of the School Psychologist in Injury Prevention, *The School Psychology Review,* 17, 1988.

Ross, J., et al, Changes in the Body Composition of Children *Journal of Physical Education, Recreation and Dance,* December 1987.

Rotatori, Anthony F. and Fox, Robert A., *Obesity in Children and Youth: Measurement, Characteristics, Causes and Treatment,* Springfield, IL, Charles C Thomas Publisher, 1989.

Saris, W. H. M., Habitual Physical Activity in Children: Methodology and Findings in Health and Disease, *Medicine and Science in Exercise and Sports,* June 1986.

Shephard, R. J., Physical Activity and "Wellness" of the Child, In R. A. Boileau, *Advances in Pediatric Sports Science, Vol. 1, Biological Issues,* Champaign, IL, *Human Kinetics,* 1984.

Siegel, J., Children's Target Heart Range, *Journal of Physical Education, Recreation and Dance,* 59, 1988.

Strong, W. B., Atherosclerosis: Its Pediatric Roots, In N. M. Kaplan and E. Stamler, (Eds.) *Prevention of Coronary Disease,* Philadelphia, W. B. Saunders, 1983.

Torun, B., Chew, F., and Mendozza, R. D., Energy Cost of Activities of Preschool Children, *Nutrition Research,* 3, 1983.

Ward, D. S. and Bar-Or, O., Role of the Physician and the Physical Education Teacher in the Treatment of Obesity at School, *Pediatrician,* 13, 1986.

Webber, L. S., et al, Tracking the Cardiovascular Disease Risk Factor Variables in School-Age Children, *Journal of Chronic Disease,* 36, 1983.

INDEX

A

Absorption, 76
ACTH, 122
Acute fatigue, 98-99
Adrenalin, 122
Adrenals, 122
Adjustment, 45
Amino acids, 78
Anger, 50
Aspirational levels, 53
Assimilation, 76
Autonomic nervous system, 44

B

Body restoration and child health, 98-117

C

Calories, 84-85
Carbohydrates, 80
Circulatory-respiratory endurance, 10
Concept of stress, 121-123
Conditioned reflex, 100
Conflict, 45
Corticoids, 122
Characteristics of childhood emotionality, 46-47
Child abuse, 124-126
Childhood obesity, 90-93
Children's eating habits, 88-90
Children's sleeping habits, 102-103
Cholesterol, 87-88
Chronic fatigue, 99

D

Daily health observation, 19
Detection and referral, 19-24
Diet, 86-88
Digestion, 76, 85-86
Dimensions of fitness, 10-13
Divorce and marital dissolution, 126-128
Dopamine, 78

E

Ears, 21-22
Elementary school health program, 137-141
Emotional arousal and reactions, 47-57
Emotional fitness, 11-12
Emotional health of children, 44-61
Emotional needs of children, 53-56
Endocrine, 122

F

Facial appearance, 20
Family relationships, 52
Fatigue, 51-52
Fats, 81
Fear, 48-49
Frustration, 45

G

General adaptation syndrome, 122
Glucose, 80
Glycogen, 80
Guidelines for emotional health of children, 56-57
Guidelines for social health of children, 67-68

H

Hair and scalp, 22
Health attitudes, 6-7

Health knowledge, 5–6
Health practice, 7–8
Health teaching, 140
Healthful school living, 139–140
Helping children learn about body restoration, 116–117
Helping children learn about emotional health, 60–62
Helping children learn about nutrition, 94–97
Helping children learn about physical activity and exercise, 42–43
Helping children learn about social health, 73–75
Helping children learn about the human organism, 24–35
Home and family stress, 123–129
Hormone, 122
Hypothalamus, 122

I

Immaturity, 45
Improving emotional health in the school environment, 57–58
Inferior health status, 52
Ingestion, 76
Intellectual fitness, 12–13
Intelligence, 12, 52
Isometric activities, 37–38
Isotonic activities, 37

J

Jealousy, 50–51
Joy, 51

L

Learning how to relax, 104–105
Life changes, 128–129

M

Maturity, 45
Meaning of fitness, 9–10
Meaning of health, 3–4
Meaning of health education, 8–9
Meaning of stress, 121

Mental practice and imagery, 112–115
Minerals, 82–83
Miscoping, 129
Muscular endurance, 10
Muscular strength, 10

N

Neurotransmitters, 76
Norepinephrine, 78
Nutrition and child health, 76–97

O

Observing emotional health, 58–60
Out-of-school physical activity programs, 40–42

P

Physical activity and exercise for children, 36
Physical characteristics of children, 15–18
Physical fitness, 9–10
Physical growth and development, 14–18
Physical health of children, 14–43
Pituitary, 122
Pleasant emotions, 11, 44
Posture, 22–23
Progressive relaxation, 105–108
Proprioceptive-facilitative activities, 36–37
Protein, 78

R

Rapid eye movements, 100
Readiness, 45
Refreshment, 103
Relaxation, 103–117
Research in social behavior, 69–71
Respiratory system, 20–21
Rest, 99

S

School health education
School health service, 137–139
School physical activity programs, 38–40
School stress, 129–136

School subjects as stressors, 133–135
Serotin, 78
Sleep, 100–120
Social distance scales, 72–73
Social environment, 52
Social fitness, 10–11
Social health of children, 63–75
Social needs of children, 63–67
Sociograms, 72
Sociographs, 72
Speech difficulties, 23–24
Status of physical fitness of children, 40–42
Stress and child health, 118–135
Stress and the child in the educative process, 130–133

T

Teacher observation of child health, 18–24

Test anxiety, 135–136
Thymus, 122
Trytophan, 78
Types of exercise for children, 36–38
Tyrosine, 78

U

Unpleasant emotions, 11, 44
Using relaxation with children, 109–112

V

Vitamins, 83

W

Water, 84
Worry, 49–50

CHARLES C THOMAS • PUBLISHER

- Hagerty, Robert—**THE CRISIS OF CONFIDENCE IN AMERICAN EDUCATION: A Blueprint for Fixing What is Wrong and Restoring America's Confidence in the Public Schools.** '95, 226 pp. (7 × 10), 1 table, $48.95, cloth, $29.95, paper.

- Morton-Young, Tommie—**AFTER-SCHOOL AND PARENT EDUCATION PROGRAMS FOR AT-RISK YOUTH AND THEIR FAMILIES: A Guide to Organizing and Operating a Community-Based Center for Basic Educational Skills Reinforcement, Homework Assistance, Cultural Enrichment, and a Parent Involvement Focus.** '95, 148 pp. (7 × 10), 1 il. Cloth—$37.95, paper—$22.95.

- Bushman, John H. & Kay Parks Bushman—**TEACHING ENGLISH CREATIVELY. (2nd Ed.)** '94, 254 pp. (7 × 10), 48 il. $47.95.

- Humphrey, James H.—**PHYSICAL EDUCATION FOR THE ELEMENTARY SCHOOL.** '94, 292 pp. (7 × 10), 8 il., $46.95. *$29.95, paper.*

- Burnsed, C. Vernon—**THE CLASSROOM TEACHER'S GUIDE TO MUSIC EDUCATION.** '93, 174 pp. (8½ × 11), 131 il., $31.95, spiral (paper).

- Clark, Lynne W.—**FACULTY AND STUDENT CHALLENGES IN FACING CULTURAL AND LINGUISTIC DIVERSITY.** '93, 282 pp. (7 × 10), 6 il., 10 tables, $51.95. *$30.95, paper.*

- Fuchs, Lucy—**HUMANITIES IN THE ELEMENTARY SCHOOL: A Handbook for Teachers.** '93, 140 pp. (7 × 10), $33.95. *$18.95, paper.*

- Mitchell, Alice Rhea—**INTERDISCIPLINARY INSTRUCTION IN READING COMPREHENSION AND WRITTEN COMMUNICATION—A Guide for An Innovative Curriculum.** '93, 110 pp. (7 × 10), $29.95. *$15.95, paper.*

- Humphrey, James H.—**STRESS MANAGEMENT FOR ELEMENTARY SCHOOLS.** '93, 198 pp. (7 × 10), $41.95. *$25.95, paper.*

- Reglin, Gary L.—**MOTIVATING LOW-ACHIEVING STUDENTS: A Special Focus on Unmotivated and Underachieving African American Students.** '93, 190 pp. (7 × 10), $45.95. *$29.95, paper.*

- Bookbinder, Robert M.—**THE PRINCIPAL: Leadership for the Effective and Productive School.** '92, 290 pp. (7 × 10), 22 il., $47.95.

- Fry, Prem S.—**FOSTERING CHILDREN'S COGNITIVE COMPETENCE THROUGH MEDIATED LEARNING EXPERIENCES: Frontiers and Futures.** '92, 358 pp. (7 × 10), $66.95. *$36.95, paper.*

- Hargis, Charles H.—**GRADES AND GRADING PRACTICES: Obstacles to Improving Education and to Helping At-Risk Students.** '90, 104 pp. (7 × 10), $23.95, paper.

- Gordon, Virginia N.—**THE UNDECIDED COLLEGE STUDENT. (2nd Ed.)** '95, 170 pp. (7 × 10), 1 il., 1 table.

- Grossman, Herbert—**EDUCATING HISPANIC STUDENTS: Implications for Instruction, Classroom Management, Counseling and Assessment. (2nd Ed.)** '95, 290 pp. (7 × 10), 17 tables, $57.95, cloth, $34.95, paper.

- Michael, Robert J.—**THE EDUCATOR'S GUIDE TO STUDENTS WITH EPILEPSY.** '95, 184 pp. (7 × 10), 5 il.

- Miller, Susan B.—**WHEN PARENTS HAVE PROBLEMS: A Book for Teens and Older Children with an Abusive, Alcoholic, or Mentally Ill Parent.** '95, 94 pp. (7 × 10), $31.95, cloth, $18.95, paper.

- Wodarski, Lois A. & John S. Wodarski.—**ADOLESCENT SEXUALITY: A Comprehensive Peer/Parent Curriculum.** '95, 168 pp. (7 × 10), 3 il., $43.95, cloth, $29.95, paper.

- Reglin, Gary L.—**AT-RISK "PARENT AND FAMILY" SCHOOL INVOLVEMENT: Strategies for Low Income Families and African-American Families of Unmotivated and Underachieving Students.** '93, 128 pp. (7 × 10), $31.95. *$16.95, paper.*

- Hawley, Peggy—**BEING BRIGHT IS NOT ENOUGH: The Unwritten Rules of Doctoral Study.** '93, 174 pp. (7 × 10), 4 il., 2 tables, $31.95, paper.

- Brigance, Albert H. & Charles H. Hargis—**EDUCATIONAL ASSESSMENT: Insuring That All Students Succeed in School.** '93, 182 pp. (7 × 10), 4 il., $39.95. *$24.95, paper.*

- Humphrey, James H.—**MOTOR LEARNING IN CHILDHOOD EDUCATION: Curricular, Compensatory, Cognitive.** '92, 206 pp. (7 × 10), $41.95. *$25.95, paper.*

- Chance, Edward W.—**VISIONARY LEADERSHIP IN SCHOOLS: Successful Strategies for Developing and Implementing an Educational Vision.** '92, 136 pp. (7 × 10), 7 il., 8 tables, $29.95. *$15.95, paper.*

- Laska, John A. & Tina Juarez—**GRADING AND MARKING IN AMERICAN SCHOOLS: Two Centuries of Debate.** '92, 162 pp. (7 × 10), $36.95. *$19.95, paper.*

- Bedwell, Lance E., Gilbert H. Hunt, Timothy J. Touzel & Dennis G. Wiseman—**EFFECTIVE TEACHING: Preparation And Implementation. (2nd Ed.)** '91, 276 pp. (7 × 10), 48 il., $39.95. *$24.95, paper.*

- Lee, Jackson F., Jr. & K. Wayne Pruitt—**PROVIDING FOR INDIVIDUAL DIFFERENCES IN STUDENT LEARNING: A Mastery Learning Approach.** '84, 130 pp., 4 il., $31.95. *$16.95, paper.*

Write, call (for Visa or MasterCard) 1-800-258-8980 or 1-217-789-8980 or FAX (217) 789-9130
Books sent on approval • Complete catalog sent on request • Prices subject to change without notice

2600 South First Street Springfield • Illinois • 62794-9265